The Lower Quadrant

A Workbook of
Manual Therapy Techniques

The Lower Quadrant
A Workbook of Manual Therapy Techniques

ISBN # 0-9736993-1-0

About the Authors

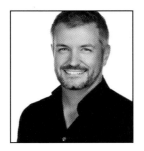

Scott Whitmore is a member of the Canadian Physiotherapy Association and a Fellow of the Canadian Academy of Manipulative Therapists. He is an instructor and examiner for the Diploma of Advanced Manual and Manipulative Therapy level system with the Orthopaedic Division of the Canadian Physiotherapy Association. He has served as Chair of the manual review committee and Chair of the education committee. Scott is owner of Manual concepts Physiotherapy in Guelph, Ontario, where he also works as a senior clinician.

www.whitmorephysiotherapy.com
www.manualconceptspt.com

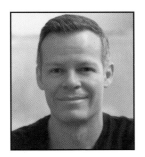

Angus Driver is a member of the Canadian Physiotherapy Association and a Fellow of the Canadian Academy of Manipulative Therapists. He is an instructor for the Diploma of Advanced Manual and Manipulative Therapy level system with the Orthopaedic Division of the Canadian Physiotherapy Association. Angus is co-owner of Adelaide West Physiotherapy in Toronto, where he also works as a senior clinician

www.adelaidewestphysiotherapy.com

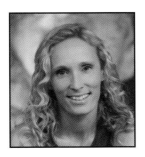

Kate Gladney is a member of the Canadian Physiotherapy Association and a Fellow of the Canadian Academy of Manipulative Therapists. She is an instructor for the Diploma of Advanced Manual and Manipulative Therapy level system with the Orthopaedic Division of the Canadian Physiotherapy Association. She is co-owner of Adelaide West Physiotherapy in Toronto, where she also works as a senior clinician

www.adelaidewestphysiotherapy.com

Acknowledgements

We would like to thank the physiotherapists who have contributed to the Canadian manual therapy system, without their hard work and dedication to the development of manual therapy techniques this book would not have be possible.

Thanks to the following people who were instrumental in getting this project completed. Greg Spadoni, Nadine Leiper, Karen Rupke, Kate Stebbings, Bev Padfield, Pary Bell, Francine Dore, Tom Gladney and Shelley Hopkins-Whitmore.

Dedication

We would like to dedicate this book to Carl Gayle. His strength of character in the face of adversity has been an inspiration to us all.

Scott, Angus, and Kate

Table of Contents

Table of Contents

List of Abbreviations

ASIS	Anterior Superior Iliac Spine
PSIS	Posterior Superior Iliac Spine
MTP	Metatarsophalangeal
IP	Interphalangeal
TMT	Tarsometatarsal
O	Stabilization
⇨	Direction of Force

The Lumbar Spine

Lumbar Spine
Active and Passive Range of Motion

Active Range of Motion

Passive Range of Motion

Passive Accessory Motion

Active Range of Motion
Flexion and Extension

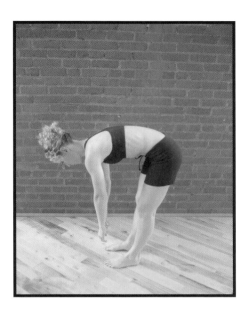
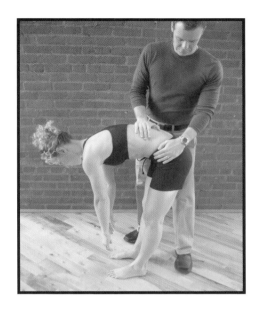

Flexion: Instruct the patient to bend forward. If the movement is pain free, stabilize the pelvis and apply overpressure. Note the range of motion, end feel and reproduction of symptoms.

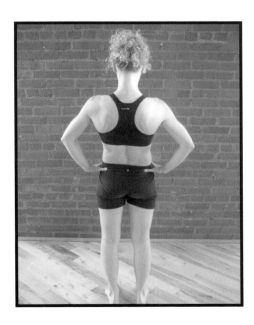
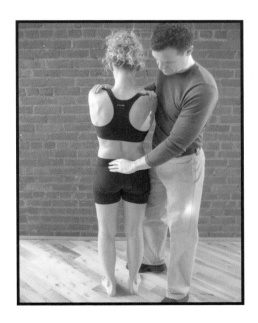

Extension: Instruct the patient to put their hands on their hips and bend backward. If the movement is pain free, stabilize the pelvis and apply overpressure. Note the range of motion, end feel and reproduction of symptoms.

Active Range of Motion
Side Flexion and Rotation

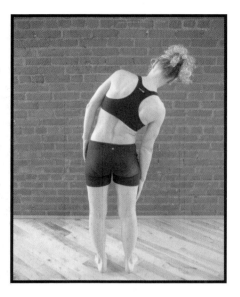
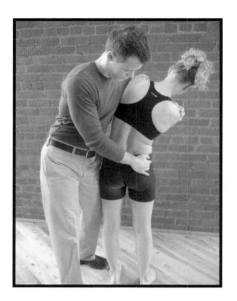

Side Flexion: Instruct the patient to bend to the right. If the movement is pain free, stabilize the pelvis and apply overpressure. Note the range of motion, end feel and reproduction of symptoms. Repeat for left side flexion.

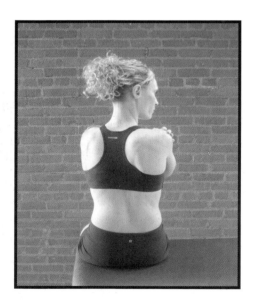
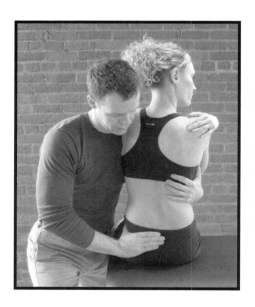

Rotation: Instruct the patient to cross their arms and twist to the right. If the movement is pain free, stabilize the pelvis and apply overpressure. Note the range of motion, end feel and reproduction of symptoms. Repeat for left rotation.

Active Range of Motion

Combined Movements

If the single plane movements in the lumbar spine are clear and you still suspect that there is a movement problem, you can use combined movements to assess the range of motion.

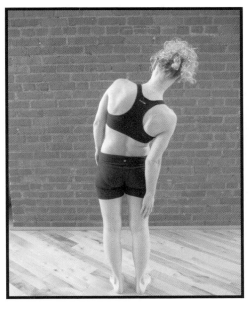 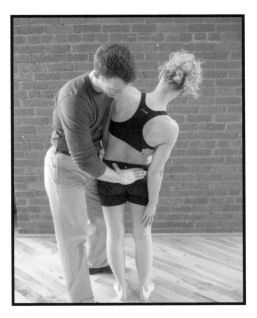

Side Flexion in Extension: Instruct the patient to bend backwards and to the right. If the movement is pain free, stabilize the pelvis and apply overpressure. Note the range of motion, end feel and reproduction of symptoms. Repeat for left side flexion in extension.

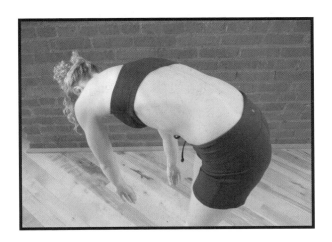 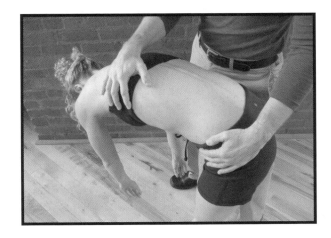

Side Flexion in Flexion: Instruct the patient to bend forward and to the right. If the movement is pain free, stabilize the pelvis and apply overpressure. Note the range of motion, end feel and reproduction of symptoms. Repeat for left side flexion in flexion.

Passive Range of Motion
Bilateral Flexion PPIVM

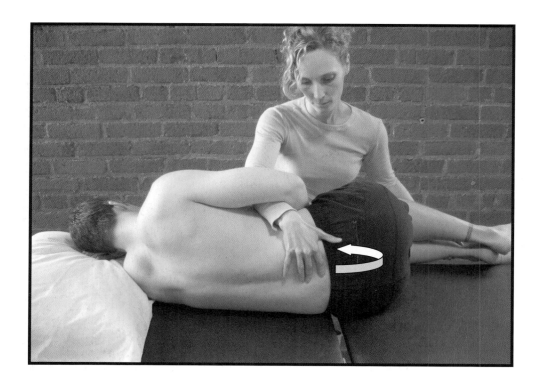

Technique described for L4-5 segment

Patient: Side lying at the edge of the bed

Therapist: Standing at the side of the bed. Support the patient's bent knees with your hip and grasp the patient's legs. Palpate the interspinous space of L4 and L5 with your index and middle fingers.

Action: Facilitate lumbar flexion by sliding the patient's legs in a cranial direction. Note the range of motion, end feel and reproduction of symptoms.

Passive Range of Motion
Bilateral Extension PPIVM

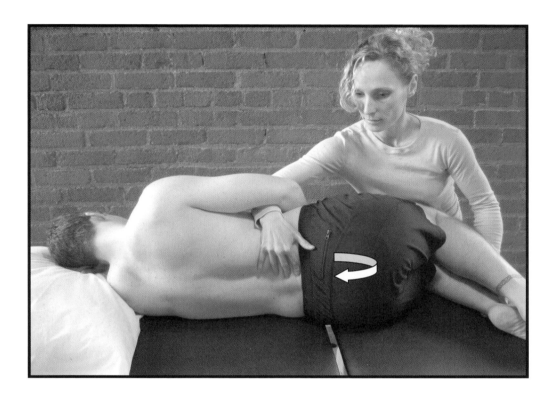

Technique described for the L4-5 segment

Patient: Side lying at the edge of the bed

Therapist: Standing at the side of the bed. Support the patient's bent knees with your hip and grasp the patient's legs. Palpate the interspinous space of L4 and L5 with your index and middle fingers.

Action: Facilitate lumbar extension by sliding the patient's legs in a posterior-caudal direction. Note the range of motion, end feel and reproduction of symptoms.

Passive Range of Motion
Unilateral Flexion PPIVM

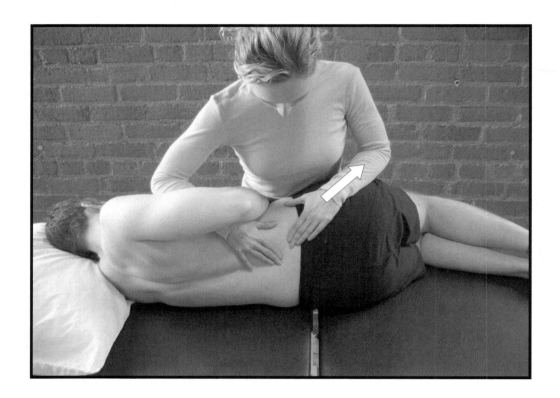

Technique described for the right L4-5 segment

Patient: Left side lying at the edge of the bed with hips flexed

Therapist: Standing at the side of the bed. Place your right arm under the patient's right arm. Palpate the transverse process of L4 with your right hand. With your left forearm on the patient's right hip, palpate the transverse process of L5 with your left hand.

Action: Facilitate unilateral flexion by applying an anterior-inferior force to L5 and the pelvis. Note the range of motion, end feel and reproduction of symptoms.

Passive Range of Motion
Unilateral Extension PPIVM

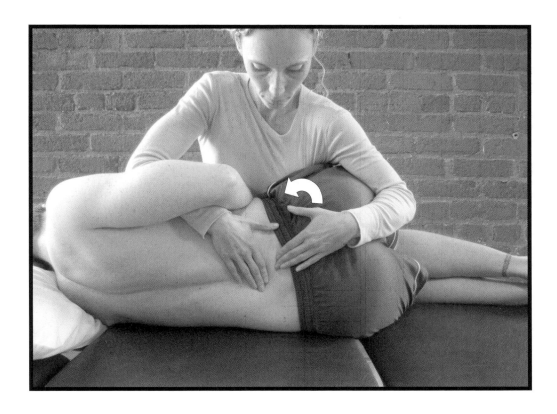

Technique described for the right L4-5 segment

Patient: Left side lying at the edge of the bed with hips flexed

Therapist: Standing at the side of the bed. Place your right arm under the patient's right arm. Palpate the transverse process of L4 with your right hand. With your left forearm on the patient's right ischial tuberosity, palpate the transverse process of L5 with your left hand.

Action: Facilitate unilateral extension by applying an anterior-superior force to L5 and the pelvis. Note the range of motion, end feel and reproduction of symptoms.

Passive Accessory Motion
Unilateral P/A Angled Cranial (Facet Joint)

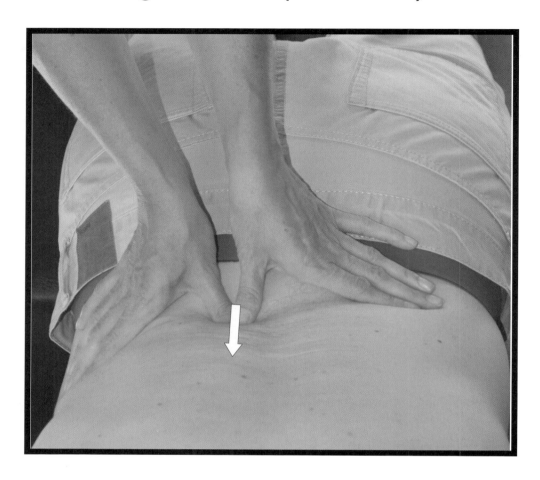

Technique described for the right L4-5 facet joint

Patient: Prone lying

Therapist: Standing at the side of the bed. Palpate the right transverse process of L4 with both thumbs.

Action: Apply a superior-anterior force to the transverse process of L4. Note the range of motion, end feel and reproduction of symptoms. This accessory motion assesses the amount of unilateral flexion at L4-5.

Passive Accessory Motion
Unilateral P/A Angled Caudal (Facet Joint)

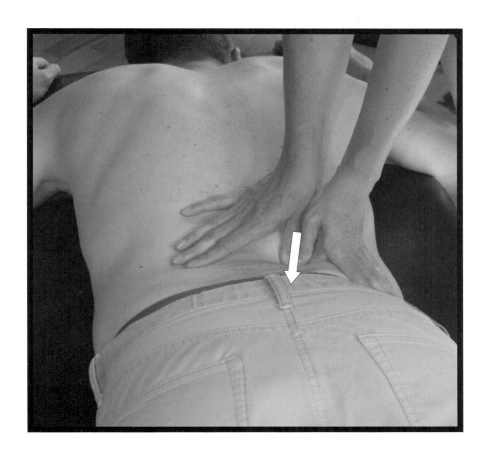

Technique described for the right L4-5 facet joint

Patient: Prone lying

Therapist: Standing at the side of the bed. Palpate the right transverse process of L4 with both thumbs.

Action: Apply a inferior-anterior force to the transverse process of L4. Note the range of motion, end feel and reproduction of symptoms. This accessory motion assesses the amount of unilateral extension at L4-5.

Lumbar Spine
Stability Testing

Stability Test
Traction

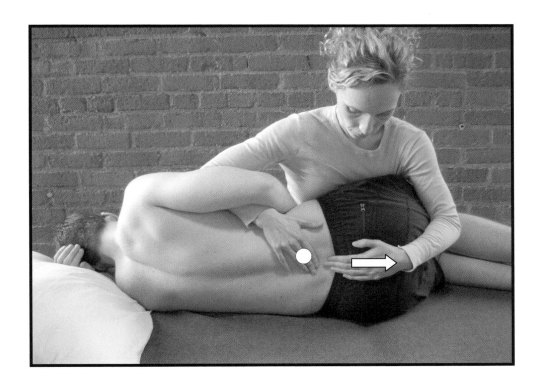

Technique described for the L4-5 segment

Patient: Side lying at the edge of the bed

Therapist: Standing at the side of the bed. Place your right arm under the patient's right arm. Stabilize the spinous process of L4 with your right hand. With your left forearm on the patient's sacrum, palpate L5 with your left hand.

Action: Apply a traction force to L5 and the pelvis. Note the end feel and reproduction of symptoms.

Stability Test
Compression

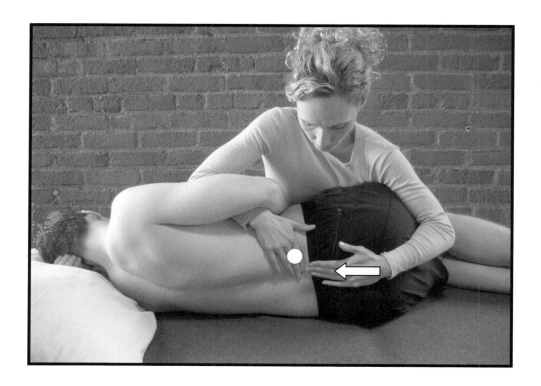

Technique described for the L4-5 segment

Patient: Side lying at the edge of the bed

Therapist: Standing at the side of the bed. Place your right arm under the patient's right arm. Stabilize the spinous process of L4 with your right hand. With your left forearm on the patient's sacrum, palpate L5 with your left hand.

Action: Apply a compression force to L5 and the pelvis. Note the end feel and reproduction of symptoms.

Stability Test
Anterior Translation

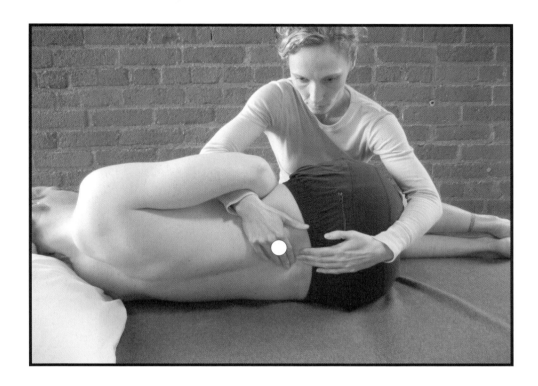

Technique described for the L4-5 segment

Patient: Side lying at the edge of the bed with hips flexed

Therapist: Standing at the side of the bed. Place your right arm under the patient's right arm. Stabilize the spinous process of L4 with your right hand. Support the patient's knees with your hip. With your left forearm on the patient's sacrum, palpate L5 with your left hand.

Action: Apply a posterior translation force to L5 by pushing the patient's legs posteriorly. This induces a relative anterior translation of L4 on L5. Note the end feel and reproduction of symptoms.

Stability Test
Posterior Translation (Dynamic Technique)

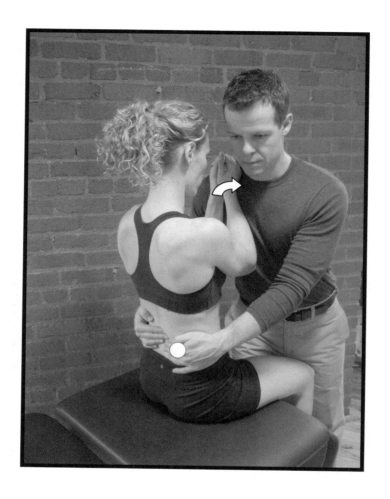

Technique described for the L4-5 segment

Patient: Sitting at the end of the bed with forearms together

Therapist: Standing at the end of the bed. Stabilize the spinous process of L5 with your left hand. Palpate the spinous process of L4 with your right hand.

Action: Instruct the patient to gently press their forearms into your upper torso. This will facilitate a contraction of the posterior paraspinal musculature inducing posterior translation of L4. Note the end feel and reproduction of symptoms.

Stability Test
Lateral Translation

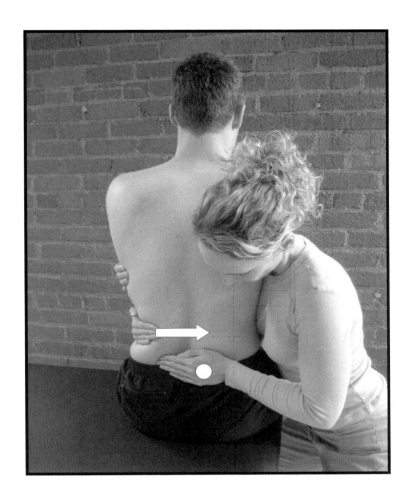

Technique described for right lateral translation of the L4-5 segment

Patient: Sitting at edge of bed with arms crossed

Therapist: Standing at the side of the bed. Place your right arm around patients trunk at the level of L4. Stabilize L5 with your left hand.

Action: Apply a right lateral translation force to L4. Note the end feel and reproduction of symptoms.

Stability Test
Torsion

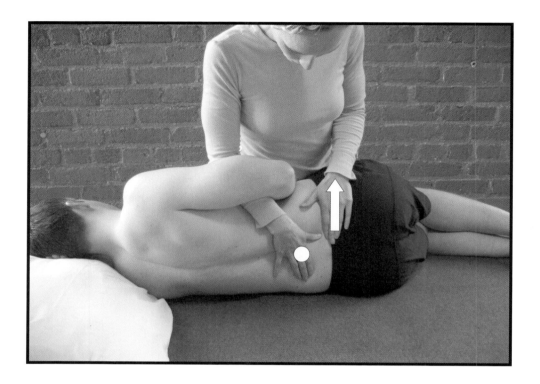

Technique described for right torsion of the L4-5 segment

Patient: Left side lying at the edge of the bed with the hips flexed

Therapist: Standing at the side of the bed. Place your right arm under the patient's right arm. Stabilize the spinous process of L4 with your right thumb. Palpate the spinous process of L5 with your left hand.

Action: Apply a left torsion force through L5 by pulling the spinous process towards the ceiling. This will induce right torsion of L4. Note the end feel and reproduction of symptoms.

Lumbar Spine
Treatment Techniques

Locking Techniques

Treatment Techniques

Locking Technique
Locking from above (Neutral)

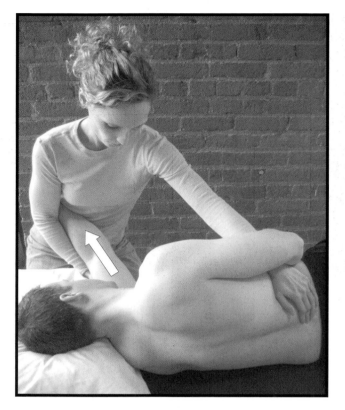

Start position

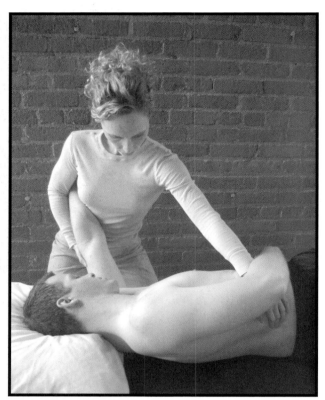

Finish position

Technique described for locking the thoracic and lumbar region to treat L4-5 in left side lying

Patient: Left side lying at the edge of the bed

Therapist: Standing at the side of the bed. Palpate the spinous process of L4 with your left hand. Grasp the patient's left arm with your right hand.

Action: Pull the patient's left arm to rotate the thorax and the lumbar spine to the right until you feel L4 start to move.

Locking Technique
Ipsilateral Locking From Above

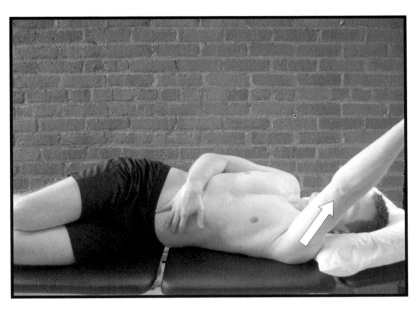

Ipsilateral side bend in extension (picture shows extension, right side flexion and right rotation)

Action: Use the same hand positions as page 20. Pull the patients left arm cranially and towards the ceiling. This will place the thorax in a position of extension, right side flexion and right rotation.

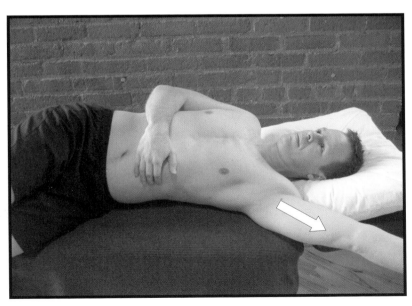

Ipsilateral side bend in flexion (picture shows flexion, right side flexion and rotation)

Action: Use the same hand positions as page 20. Pull the patients left arm cranially and parallel to the floor. This will place the thorax in a position of flexion, right side flexion and right rotation.

Locking Technique
Contralateral Locking From Above

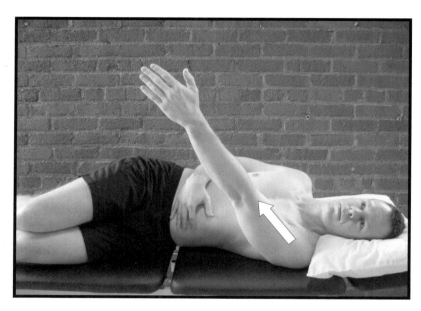

Contralateral side bend in extension (picture shows extension, left side flexion and right rotation)

Action: Use the same hand positions as page 20. Pull the patients left arm caudally and towards the ceiling. This will place the thorax in a position of extension, left side flexion and right rotation.

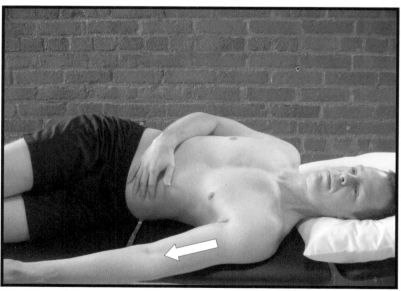

Contralateral side bend in flexion (picture shows flexion, left side flexion and right rotation)

Action: Use the same hand positions as page 20. Pull the patients arm caudally and parallel to the floor. This will place the thorax in a position of flexion, left side flexion and right rotation.

Locking Technique
Locking From Below

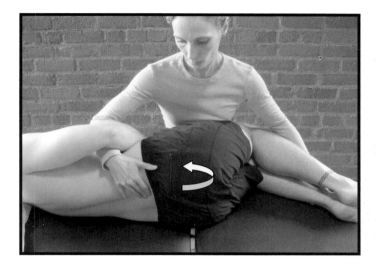

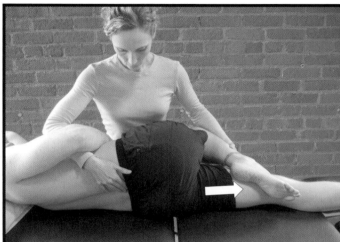

Start position   **Finish position**

Technique described for locking the lumbar region in flexion to treat L4-5 in left side lying

Patient: Left side lying at the edge of the bed with hips flexed

Therapist: Standing at the side of the bed. Place your right arm under the patient's right arm. Palpate the spinous process of L5 with your right hand. Grasp the patient's legs with your left hand.

Action: Slide the patient's legs in a cranial direction and stop once you feel the spinous process of L5 start to move. Hold onto the patient's right leg and instruct the patient to straighten their left leg. Place their right foot behind their left knee. Bilateral extension can also be utilized to lock the lower segments.

Treatment Technique
Traction

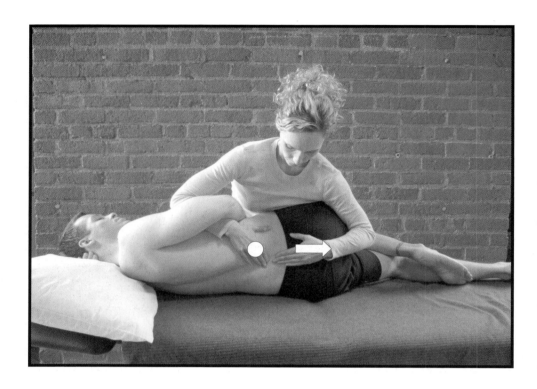

Technique described for the L4-5 segment with the patient in left side lying

Indication: Articular restriction of the lumbar spine

Patient: Left side lying close to the edge of bed

Therapist: Standing at the side of the bed. Lock the patient from above and below, leaving L4-5 in neutral. Place your right arm under the patient's right arm. Stabilize the spinous process of L4 with your right hand. With your left forearm on the patient's sacrum, palpate L5 with your left hand.

Action: Apply a traction force to L5 and the pelvis. This technique can be graded from 1 to 4.

Treatment Technique
Unilateral Flexion
Direct Technique

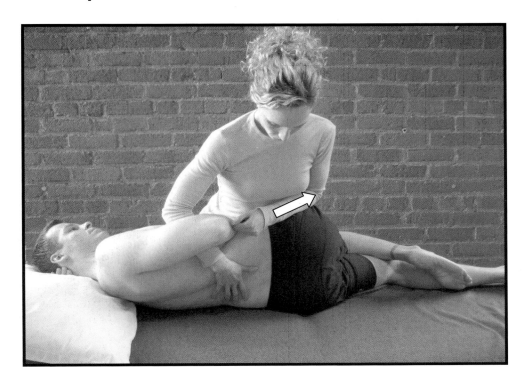

Technique described for the right L4-5 facet joint

Indication: Unilateral articular restriction of flexion

Patient: Left side lying at the edge of the bed

Therapist: Standing at the side of the bed. Lock the patient from above and below, leaving L4-5 in neutral. Place your right arm under the patient's right arm and stabilize it against the thorax with your right hip. Palpate the spinous process of L4 with your right hand. Place your left forearm on the patient's iliac crest.

Action: Apply an anterior-inferior force to the patient's pelvis. This technique can be graded from 1 to 4. Active mobilization can be utilized by instructing the patient to meet the therapists resistance at the motion barrier. Resist the direction which facilitates further left side flexion and right rotation. Hold the contraction for 5 seconds and then take up the new motion barrier. Repeat this process 3 times and then reassess your active and passive movement tests.

Treatment Technique
Unilateral Flexion
Indirect Technique

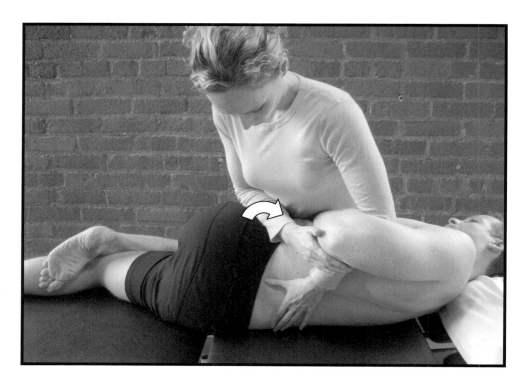

Technique described for the right L4-5 facet joint

Indication: Unilateral articular restriction of flexion

Patient: Right side lying at the edge of the bed

Therapist: Standing at the side of the bed. Lock into the L4-5 segment using contralateral flexion from above and flexion from below. Place your left arm under the patient's left arm and stabilize it against the patient's thorax with your left hip. Palpate the spinous process of L4 with your left hand. Place your right forearm on the patient's iliac crest.

Action: Apply a superior-anterior force to the patient's pelvis. This will induce flexion, left side flexion and left rotation at the right L4-5 facet joint. This technique can be graded from 1 to 4. Active mobilization can be utilized by instructing the patient to meet the therapists resistance at the motion barrier. Resist the direction which facilitates further left side flexion and left rotation. Hold the contraction for 5 seconds and then take up the new motion barrier. Repeat this process 3 times and then reassess your active and passive movement tests.

Treatment Techniques
Unilateral Extension
Direct Technique

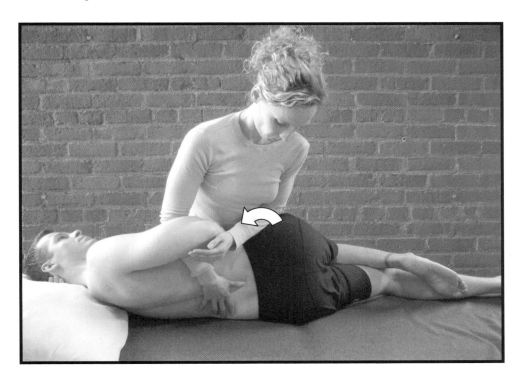

Technique described for the right L4-5 facet joint

Indication: Unilateral articular restriction of extension

Patient: Left side lying at the edge of the bed

Therapist: Standing at the side of the bed. Lock the patient from above and below, leaving L4-5 in neutral. Place your right arm under the patient's right arm and stabilize it against the patient's thorax with your right hip. Palpate the spinous process of L4 with your right hand. Place your left forearm on the patient's iliac crest.

Action: Apply a superior-anterior force to the patient's pelvis. This technique can be graded from 1 to 4.

Active mobilization can be utilized by instructing the patient to meet the therapists resistance at the motion barrier. Resist the direction which facilitates further right side flexion and right rotation. Hold the contraction for 5 seconds and then take up the new motion barrier. Repeat this process 3 times and then reassess your active and passive movement tests.

Treatment Techniques
Unilateral Extension
Indirect Technique

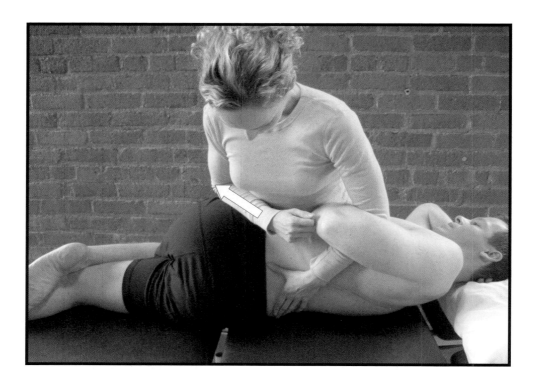

Technique described for the right L4-5 facet joint

Indication: Unilateral articular restriction of extension

Patient: Right side lying at the edge of the bed

Therapist: Standing at the side of the bed. Lock into the L4-5 segment using contralateral extension from above and extension from below. Place your left arm under the patient's left arm and stabilize it against the patient's thorax with your left hip. Palpate the spinous process of L4 with your left hand. Place your right forearm on the patient's iliac crest.

Action: Apply an anterior-inferior force to the patient's pelvis. This will induce extension, right side flexion and left rotation at the right L4-5 facet joint. This technique can be graded from 1 to 4. Active mobilization can be utilized by instructing the patient to meet the therapists resistance at the motion barrier. Resist the direction which facilitates further right side flexion and left rotation. Hold the contraction for 5 seconds and then take up the new motion barrier. Repeat this process 3 times and then reassess your active and passive movement tests.

Treatment Technique
Unilateral Flexion
Superior-Anterior Glide

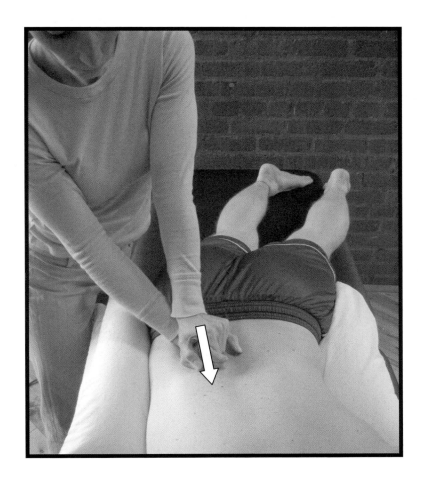

Technique described for the right L4-5 facet joint

Indication: Unilateral articular restriction of flexion

Patient: Prone lying over a pillow in the restricted position of lumbar left side flexion

Therapist: Standing at the side of the bed. Place the pisiform of your right hand over the right transverse process of L4. Overlap your right hand with your left hand.

Action: Apply a superior-anterior glide to the transverse process of L4. This technique can be graded from 1 to 4.

Treatment Technique
Unilateral Extension
Posterior-Inferior Glide

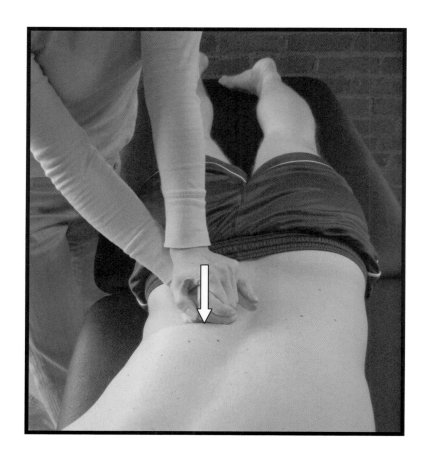

Technique described for the right L4-5 facet joint

Indication: Unilateral articular restriction of extension

Patient: Prone lying in the restricted position of lumbar right side flexion

Therapist: Standing at the side of the bed. Place the pisiform of your right hand over the right transverse process of L5. Overlap your right hand with your left hand.

Action: Apply a superior-anterior glide to the transverse process of L5. This will facilitate a relative posterior-inferior glide of the right L4-L5 facet joint. This technique can be graded from 1 to 4.

The Thoracolumbar Junction

Thoracolumbar Junction
Active and Passive Range of Motion

Active Range of Motion
Flexion and Extension

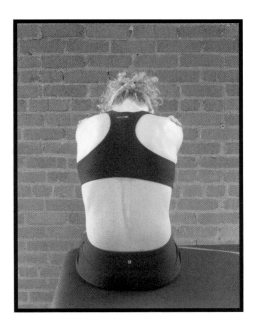 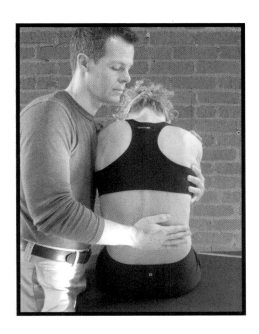

Flexion: Patient sitting at the end of the bed with their arms crossed. Instruct the patient to bend forward. If the movement is pain free, stabilize L1 and apply overpressure. Note the range of motion, end feel and reproduction of symptoms.

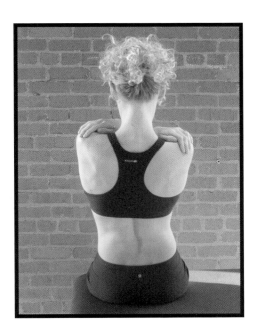 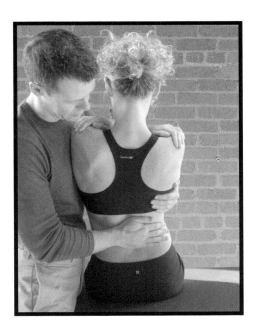

Extension: Patient sitting at the end of the bed with their arms crossed. Instruct the patient to bend backward. If the movement is pain free, stabilize L1 and apply overpressure. Note the range of motion, end feel and reproduction of symptoms.

Active Range of Motion
Side Flexion and Rotation

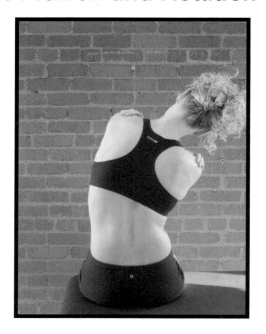 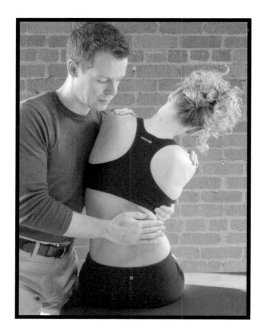

Side Flexion: Patient sitting at the end of the bed with their arms crossed. Instruct the patient to bend to the right. If the movement is pain free, stabilize L1 and apply overpressure. Note the range of motion, end feel and reproduction of symptoms. Repeat for left side flexion.

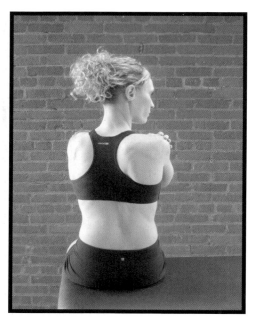 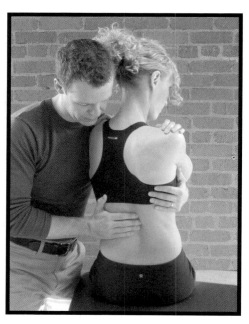

Rotation: Patient sitting at the end of the bed with their arms crossed. Instruct the patient to twist to the right. If the movement is pain free, stabilize L1 and apply overpressure. Note the range of motion, end feel and reproduction of symptoms. Repeat for left rotation.

Active Range of Motion
Combined Movements

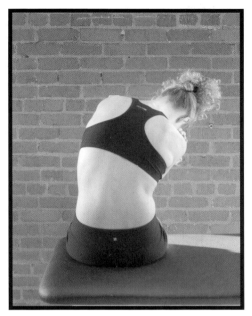 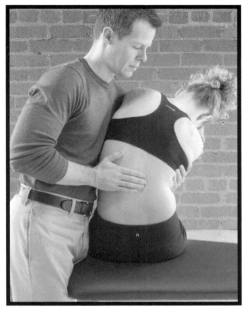

Right side flexion in flexion: Patient sitting at the end of the bed with their arms crossed. Instruct the patient to bend forward and to the right. If the movement is pain free, stabilize L1 and apply overpressure. Note the range of motion, end feel and reproduction of symptoms. Repeat for left side flexion in flexion.

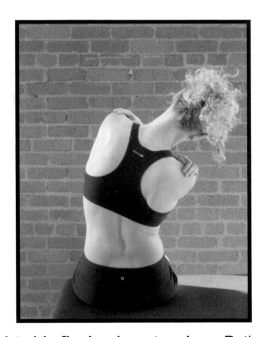 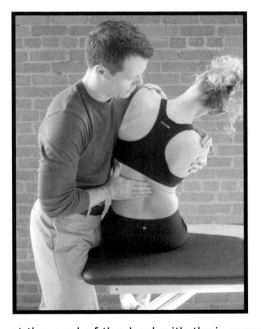

Right side flexion in extension: Patient sitting at the end of the bed with their arms crossed. Instruct the patient to bend backward and to the right. If the movement is pain free, stabilize L1 and apply overpressure. Note the range of motion, end feel and reproduction of symptoms. Repeat for left side flexion in extension.

Passive Range of Motion
Bilateral Flexion PPIVM

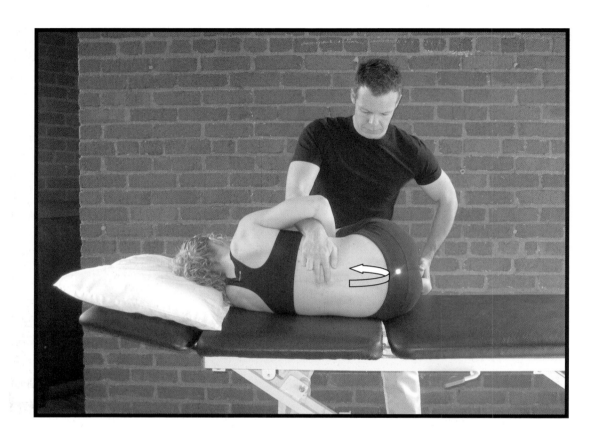

Technique described for T12-L1 segment

Patient: Side lying at the edge of the bed

Therapist: Standing at the side of the bed. Support the patient's bent knees with your hip and grasp the patient's legs. Palpate the interspinous space of T12 and L1 with your index and middle fingers.

Action: Facilitate flexion by sliding the patient's legs in a cranial direction. Note the range of motion, end feel and reproduction of symptoms.

Passive Range of Motion
Bilateral Extension PPIVM

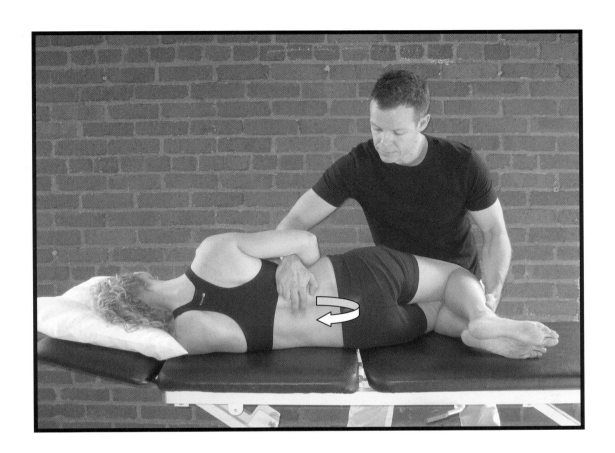

Technique described for T12-L1 segment

Patient: Side lying at the edge of the bed

Therapist: Standing at the side of the bed. Support the patient's bent knees with your hip and grasp the patient's legs. Palpate the interspinous space of T12 and L1 with your index and middle fingers.

Action: Facilitate extension by sliding the patient's legs in a posterior- caudal direction. Note the range of motion, end feel and reproduction of symptoms.

Passive Range of Motion
Unilateral Flexion / Extension PPIVM

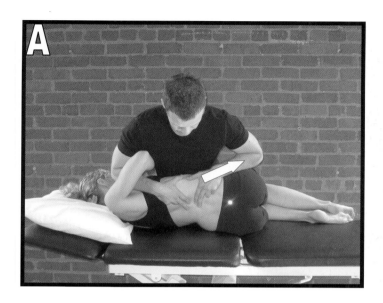 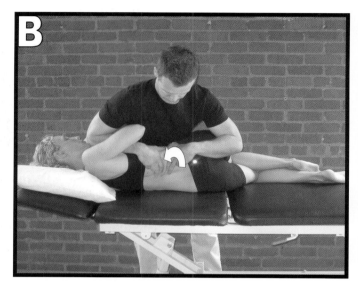

Technique described for T12 - L1 segment

Patient: Side lying at the edge of the bed

Therapist: Standing at the side of the bed. Place your right arm under the patient's right arm. Palpate the transverse process of T12 with your right hand. With your left forearm on the patient's right hip, palpate the transverse process of L1 with your left hand.

Action: Facilitate unilateral flexion by applying an anterior-inferior force to L1 and the pelvis. Note the range of motion, end feel and reproduction of symptoms.

Repeat as above, for unilateral extension by applying an anterior-superior force to L1 and the pelvis. Note the range of motion, end feel and reproduction of symptoms.(B).

Passive Accessory Motion
Posterior Anterior Pressure Angled Cranial (Facet Joint)

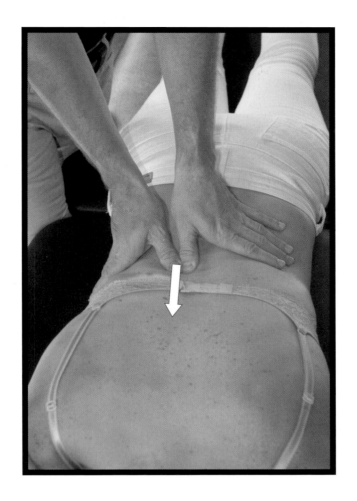

Technique described for the right T12-L1 facet joint

Patient: Prone lying

Therapist: Standing at the side of the bed. Palpate the right transverse process of T12 with both thumbs.

Action: Apply a superior-anterior force to the transverse process of T12. Note the range of motion, end feel and reproduction of symptoms. This accessory motion assesses the amount of unilateral flexion at T12-L1.

Passive Accessory Motion
Posterior Anterior Pressure Angled Caudal (Facet Joint)

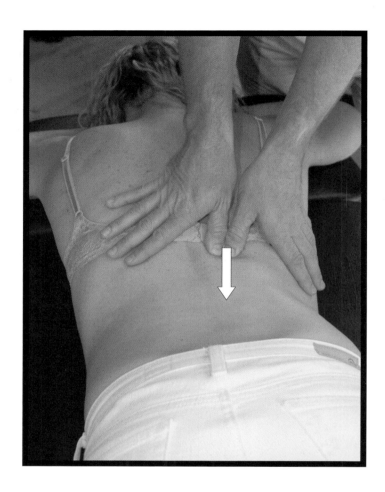

Technique described for the right T12-L1 facet joint

Patient: Prone lying

Therapist: Standing at the side of the bed. Palpate the right transverse process of T12 with both thumbs.

Action: Apply an anterior-inferior force to the transverse process of T12. Note the range of motion, end feel and reproduction of symptoms. This accessory motion assesses the amount of unilateral extension at T12-L1.

Thoracolumbar Junction
Stability Testing

Stability Test
Traction

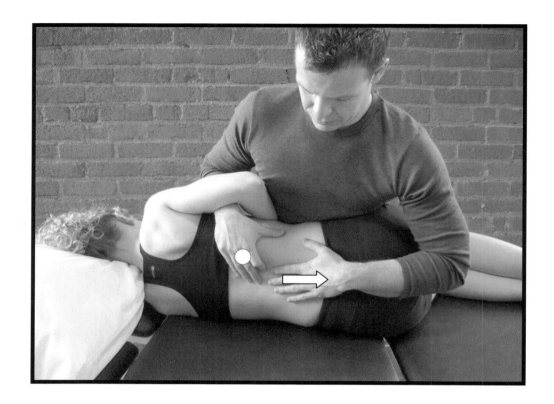

Technique described for the T12-L1 segment

Patient: Side lying at the edge of the bed

Therapist: Standing at the side of the bed. Place your right arm under the patient's right arm. Stabilize the spinous process of T12 with your right hand. With your left forearm on the patient's sacrum, palpate L1 with your left hand.

Action: Apply a traction force to the lumbar spine and pelvis. Note the end feel and reproduction of symptoms.

Stability Test
Compression

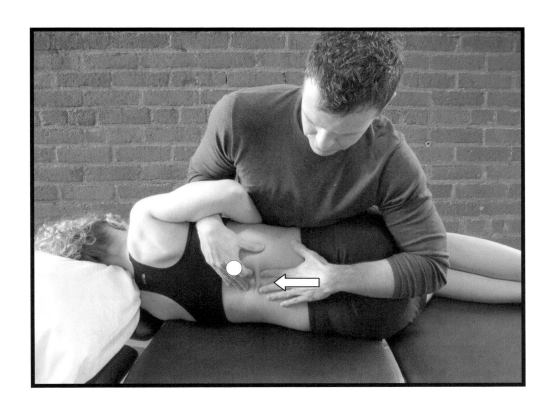

Technique described for the T12-L1 segment

Patient: Side lying at the edge of the bed

Therapist: Standing at the side of the bed. Place your right arm under the patient's right arm. Stabilize the spinous process of T12 with your right hand. With your left forearm on the patient's sacrum, palpate L1 with your left hand.

Action: Apply a compression force to the lumbar spine and pelvis. Note the end feel and reproduction of symptoms.

Stability Test
Anterior Translation

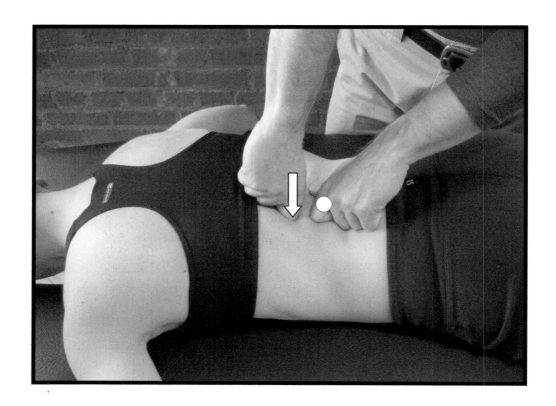

Technique described for the T12-L1 segment

Patient: Prone lying

Therapist: Standing at the side of the bed. With your left hand, stabilize L1 with a key grip. Palpate the transverse processes of T12 with your right hand using a key grip.

Action: Apply an anterior translation force to T12. Note the end feel and reproduction of symptoms.

Stability Test
Posterior Translation

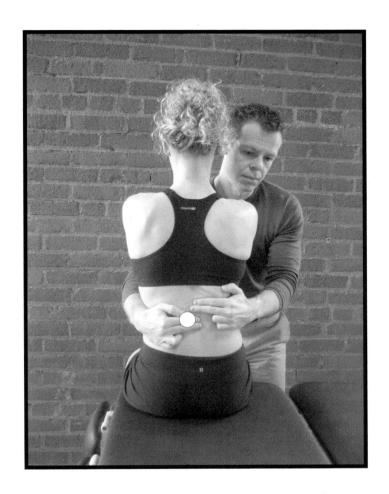

Technique described for the T12-L1 segment

Patient: Sitting at the end of the bed with forearms together

Therapist: Standing at the end of the bed. Stabilize the spinous process of L1 with your right hand. Palpate the spinous process of T12 with your left hand.

Action: Instruct the patient to gently press their forearms into your upper torso. This will facilitate a contraction of the posterior paraspinal musculature inducing posterior translation of T12. Note the end feel and reproduction of symptoms.

Stability Test
Lateral Translation

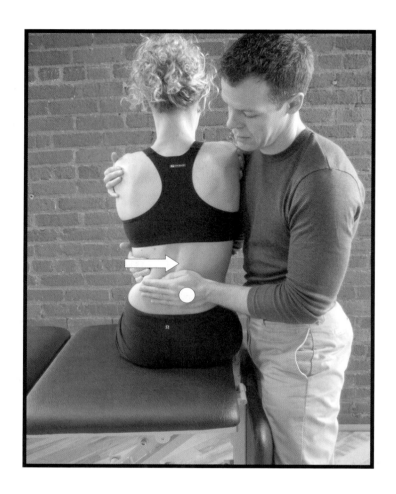

Technique described for right lateral translation of the T12-L1 segment

Patient: Sitting at edge of bed with arms crossed

Therapist: Standing at the side of the bed. Place your right arm around patients trunk at the level of T12. Stabilize L1 with your left hand.

Action: Apply a right lateral translation force to T12. Note the end feel and reproduction of symptoms.

Stability Test
Torsion

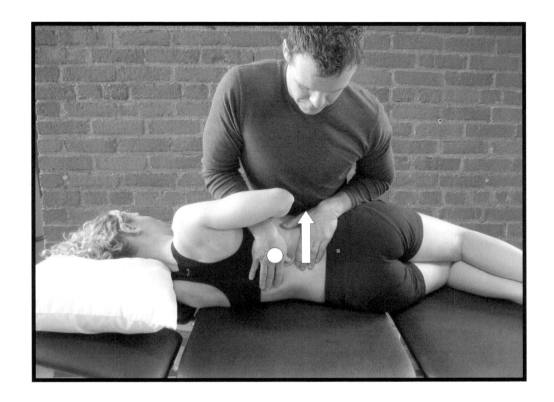

Technique described for right torsion of the T12-L1 segment

Patient: Left side lying at the edge of the bed with the hips flexed

Therapist: Standing at the side of the bed. Place your right arm under the patient's right arm. Stabilize the spinous process of T12 with your right thumb. Palpate the spinous process of L1 with your left hand.

Action: Apply a left torsion force through L1 by pulling the spinous process towards the ceiling. This will induce right torsion of T12. Note the end feel and reproduction of symptoms.

Thoracolumbar Junction
Treatment Techniques

Treatment Technique
Traction

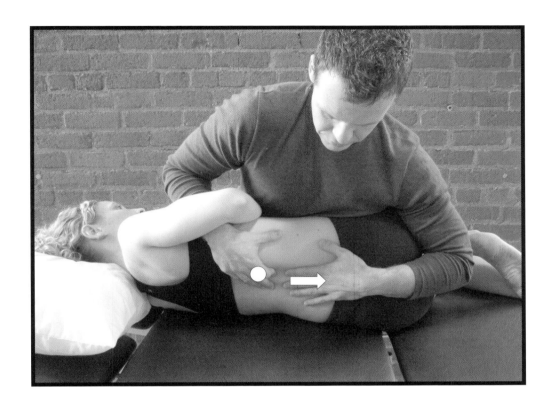

Technique described for the T12-L1 segment in left side lying

Indication: Articular restriction

Patient: Left side lying close to the edge of bed

Therapist: Standing at the side of the bed. Lock the patient from above and below, leaving T12-L1 in neutral. Place your right arm under the patient's right arm. Stabilize the spinous process of T12 with your right hand. With your left forearm on the patient's sacrum, palpate L1 with your left hand.

Action: Apply a traction force to the lumbar spine and pelvis. This technique can be graded from 1 to 4.

Treatment Technique
Unilateral Flexion
(Direct Technique)

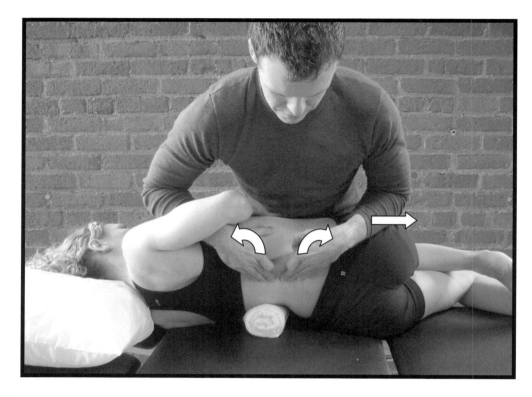

Technique described for the right T12-L1 facet joint

Indication: Unilateral articular restriction of flexion

Patient: Left side lying at the edge of the bed with a rolled towel placed under the T12-L1 segment

Therapist: Standing at the side of the bed. Lock the patient from above and below, leaving T12-L1 in neutral. Place your right arm under the patient's right arm and stabilize it against the thorax with your right hip. Palpate the spinous process of T12 with your right hand. Place your left forearm on the patient's iliac crest and palpate the spinous process of L1.

Action: Apply an inferior force through the patient's pelvis with your left forearm while facilitating left side flexion with your hands. This technique can be graded from 1 to 4. Active mobilization can be utilized by instructing the patient to meet the therapists resistance at the motion barrier. Resist the direction which facilitates further left side flexion. Hold the contraction for 5 seconds and then take up the new motion barrier. Repeat this process 3 times and then reassess your active and passive movement tests.

Treatment Technique
Unilateral Extension
(Indirect Technique)

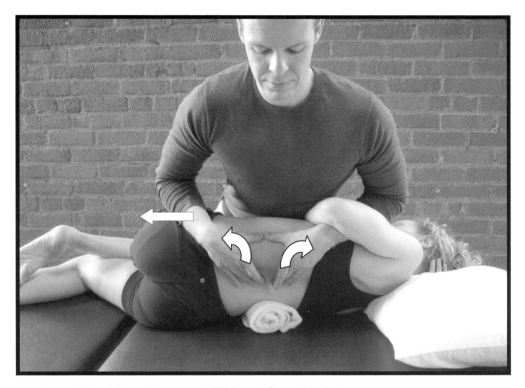

Technique described for the right T12-L1 facet joint

Indication: Unilateral articular restriction of extension

Patient: Right side lying at the edge of the bed with a rolled towel placed under the T12-L1 segment

Therapist: Standing at the side of the bed. Lock into the T12-L1 segment using contralateral extension from above and extension from below. Place your left arm under the patient's left arm and stabilize it against the patient's thorax with your left hip. Palpate the spinous process of T12 with your left hand. Place your right forearm on the patient's iliac crest and palpate the spinous process of L1.

Action: Apply an inferior force through the patient's pelvis with your right forearm while facilitating right side flexion with your hands. This technique can be graded from 1 to 4. Active mobilization can be utilized by instructing the patient to meet the therapists resistance at the motion barrier. Resist the direction which facilitates further right side flexion. Hold the contraction for 5 seconds and then take up the new motion barrier. Repeat this process 3 times and then reassess your active and passive movement tests.

The Pelvis

The Pelvis © 2005

The Pelvis
Active and Passive Range of Motion

Active Range of Motion

Passive Range of Motion

Passive Accessory Motion

Active Range of Motion
Habitual Movements
Forward and Backward Bending

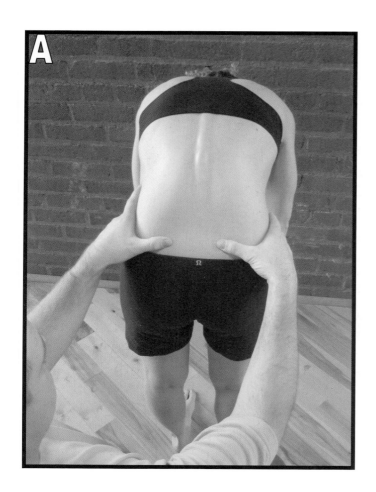

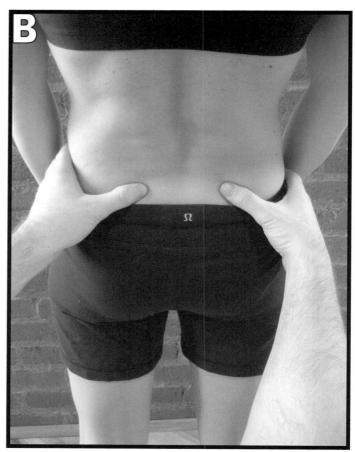

Patient: Standing

Therapist: Crouching behind the patient. Place your right thumb on the patient's right PSIS and your left thumb on the patient's left PSIS.

Action: Instruct the patient to move through forward bending (A) and backward bending (B). Observe the movement between the patient's two innominates. Asymmetry of movement may indicate SI joint dysfunction and requires further assessment.

Active Range of Motion
Habitual Movements
Side Flexion and Rotation

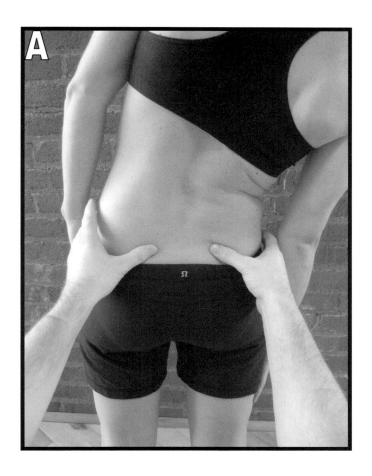 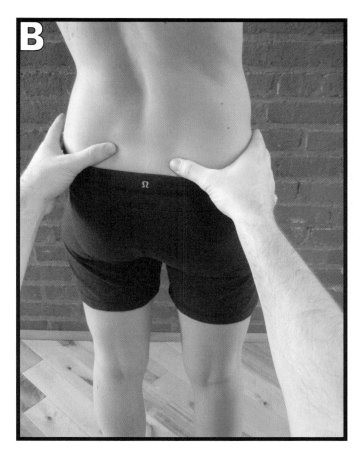

Patient: Standing

Therapist: Crouching behind the patient. Place your right thumb on the patient's right PSIS and your left thumb on the patient's left PSIS.

Action: Instruct the patient to move through right side flexion (A) or right rotation (B). Observe the movement between the patient's two innominates. Asymmetry of movement may indicate SI joint dysfunction and requires further assessment. Repeat for left side flexion and left rotation.

Active Range of Motion
Standing Flexion Kinetic Test

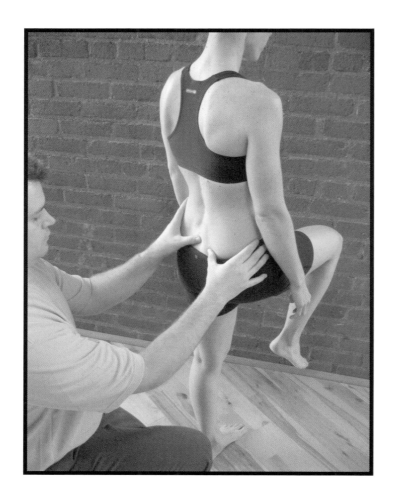

Technique described for the right SI joint

Patient: Standing

Therapist: Crouching behind the patient. Place your right thumb on the patient's right PSIS and your left thumb on the spinous process of S2.

Action: Instruct the patient to flex their right hip. Observe the movement between the right PSIS and the sacrum. Asymmetry of movement may indicate SI joint dysfunction and requires further assessment.

Active Range of Motion
Standing Extension Kinetic Test

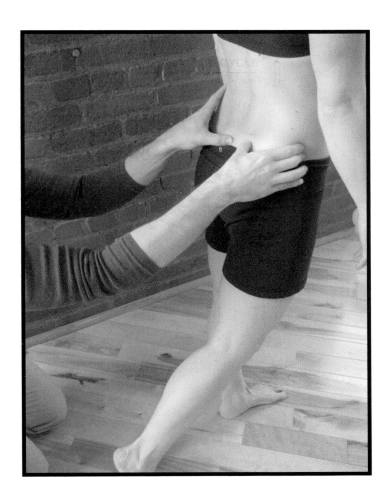

Technique described for the right SI joint

Patient: Standing

Therapist: Crouching behind the patient. Place your right thumb on the patient's right PSIS and the left thumb on the spinous process of S2.

Action: Instruct the patient to extend the right hip. Observe the movement between the right PSIS and the sacrum. Asymmetry of movement may indicate SI joint dysfunction and requires further assessment.

Active Range of Motion
Standing Contralateral Kinetic Test

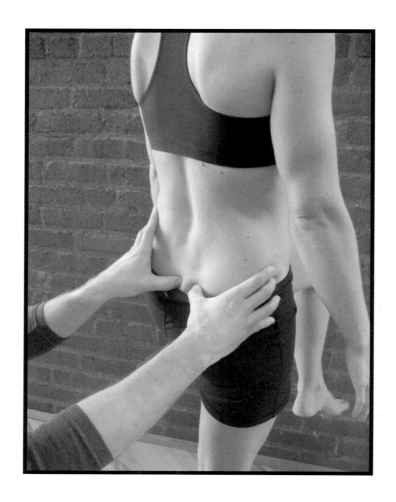

Technique described for the right SI joint

Patient: Standing

Therapist: Crouching behind the patient. Place your right thumb on the patient's right PSIS and the left thumb on the spinous process of S2

Action: Instruct the patient to flex the left hip. Observe the movement between the right PSIS and the sacrum. Asymmetry of movement may indicate SI joint dysfunction and requires further assessment.

Passive Range of Motion
Innominate Anterior Rotation

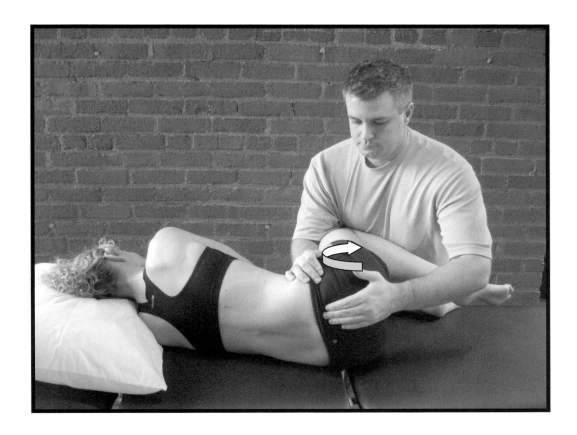

Technique described for the right SI joint

Patient: Left side lying at the edge of the bed with hips flexed

Therapist: Standing at the side of the bed. Flex the patient's top leg and place it on your abdomen. Place your right hand on the patient's right ASIS. Place your left hand on the patient's right PSIS.

Action: Passively rotate the innominate anteriorly. Note the range of motion, end feel and reproduction of symptoms.

Passive Range of Motion
Innominate Posterior Rotation

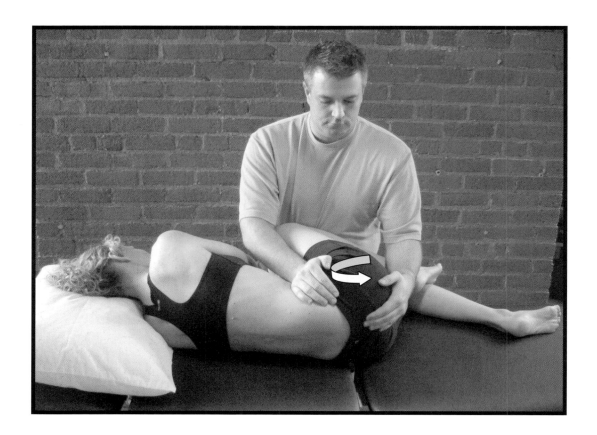

Technique described for the right SI joint

Patient: Left side lying at the edge of the bed with hips flexed

Therapist: Standing at the side of the bed. Flex the patient's top leg and place it on your abdomen. Place the heel of your right hand on the patient's right ASIS. Place your left hand on the patient's right ischial tuberosity.

Action: Passively rotate the innominate posteriorly. Note the range of motion, end feel and reproduction of symptoms.

Passive Range of Motion
Sacrum Nutation

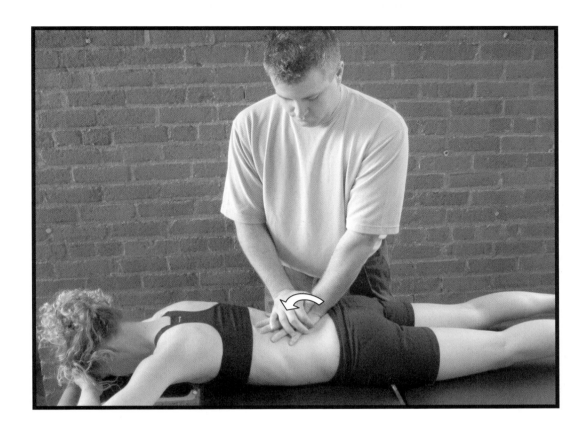

Patient: Prone lying

Therapist: Standing at the side of the bed. Place the palm of your left hand on the base of the sacrum and overlap with the right hand.

Action: Apply an anterior directed force to the base of the sacrum to induce nutation. Note the range of motion, end feel and reproduction of symptoms.

Passive Range of Motion
Sacrum Counternutation

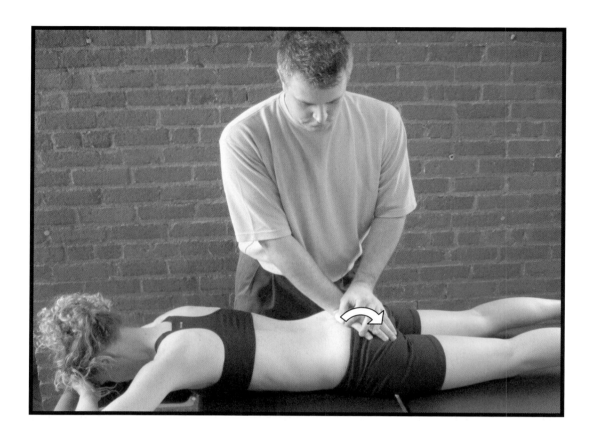

Patient: Prone lying

Therapist: Standing at the side of the bed. Place the palm of your right hand on the apex of the sacrum and overlap with your left hand.

Action: Apply an anterior directed force to the apex of the sacrum to induce counternutation. Note the range of motion, end feel and reproduction of symptoms.

Passive Accessory Motion
Innominate Inferior-Posterior Glide

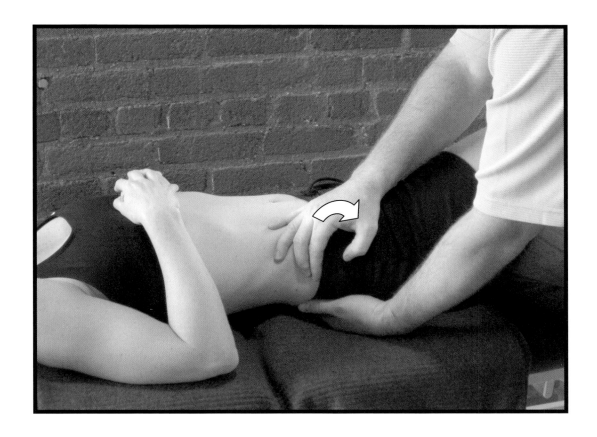

Technique described for the right SI joint

Patient: Supine lying with knee flexed over a roll or the therapist's leg

Therapist: Standing at the side of the bed. Palpate the right sacral sulcus and spinous process of L5 with the left middle and index finger respectively. Place the heel of your right hand over the right ASIS .

Action: Passively rotate the right innominate through anterior rotation. The end of the motion is reached when L5 begins to move. This will induce an inferior-posterior glide of the innominate on the sacrum. Note the range of motion, end feel and reproduction of symptoms.

Passive Accessory Motion
Innominate Anterior-Superior Glide

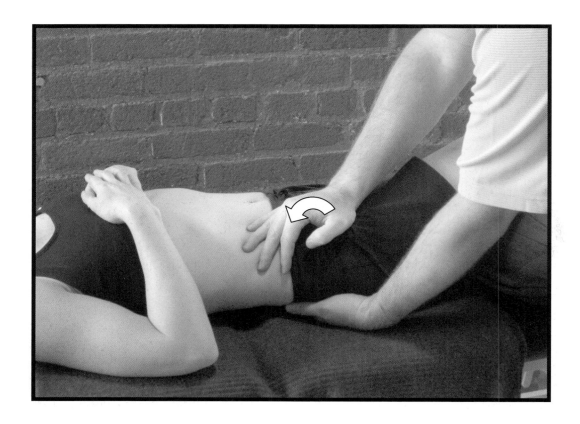

Technique described for the right SI joint

Patient: Supine lying with knee flexed over a roll or the therapist's leg

Therapist: Standing at the side of the bed. Palpate the right sacral sulcus and spinous process of L5 with the left middle and index finger respectively. Place the heel of your right hand over the right ASIS .

Action: Passively rotate the right innominate posteriorly. The end of the motion is reached when L5 begins to move. This will induce a superior-anterior glide of the innominate on the sacrum. Note the range of motion, end feel and reproduction of symptoms.

Passive Accessory Motion
Sacrum Inferior-Posterior Glide

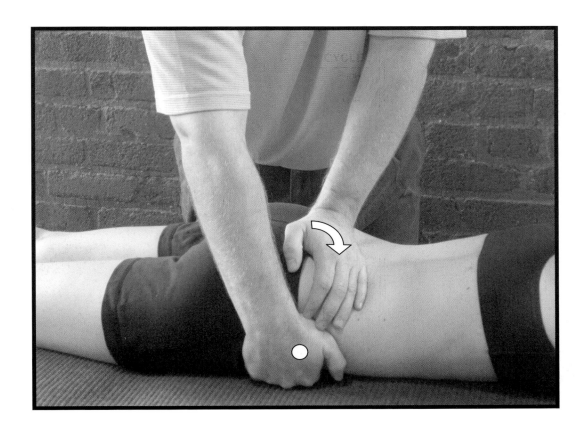

Technique described for the right SI joint

Patient: Prone lying

Therapist: Standing at the side of the bed. Stabilize the right ASIS with your right hand. Place the ulnar border of your left hand on the right sacral base.

Action: Passively nutate the right sacral base. This will induce an inferior-posterior glide of the sacrum on the innominate. Note the range of motion, end feel and reproduction of symptoms.

Passive Accessory Motion
Sacrum Anterior-Superior Glide

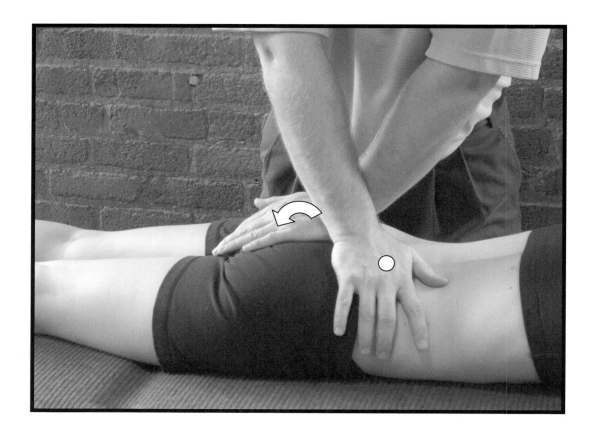

Technique described for the right SI joint

Patient: Prone lying

Therapist: Standing at the side of the bed. Stabilize the right PSIS with your right hand. Place the ulnar border of your left hand on the apex of the sacrum

Action: Passively counternutate the right sacral base. This will induce a superior-anterior glide of the sacrum on the innominate. Note the range of motion, end feel and reproduction of symptoms.

The Pelvis
Stability Testing

Joint Stability Tests

Ligament Stress Tests

Stability Test
Posterior Translation

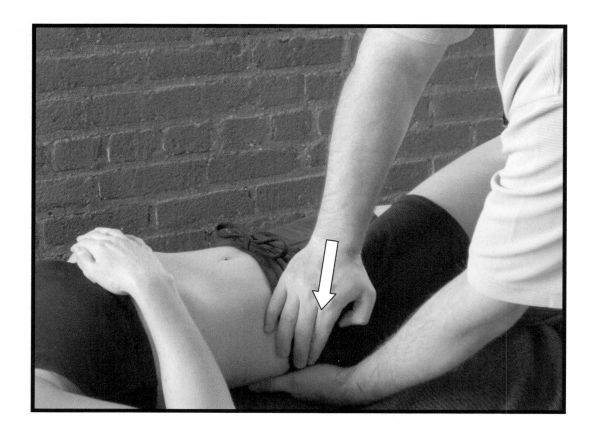

Technique described for the right SI joint

Patient: Supine lying with knee flexed over a roll or the therapist's leg

Therapist: Standing at the side of the bed. Palpate the right sacral sulcus and the spinous process of L5 with the left middle and index finger respectively. Place the heel of your right hand over the right ASIS .

Action: Apply a posterior translation force to the innominate. The end of the motion is reached when L5 begins to move. Note the end feel and reproduction of symptoms.

Stability Test
Superior Translation

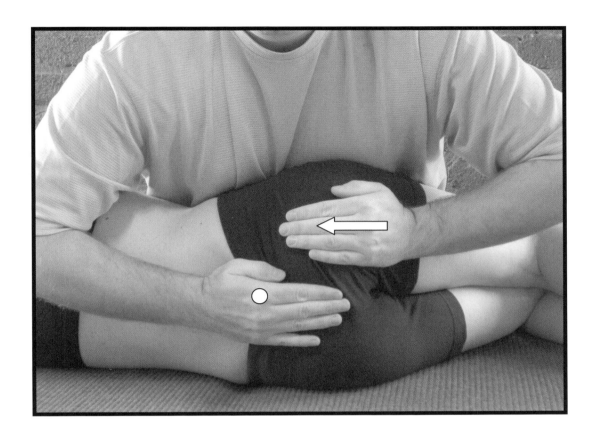

Technique described for the right SI joint

Patient: Left side lying with hips flexed

Therapist: Standing at the side of the bed. Stabilize the sacrum with the heel of your right hand. Palpate the right ischial tuberosity with the heel of your left hand.

Action: Apply a superior translation force to the ischial tuberosity. Note the end feel and reproduction of symptoms.

Stability Test
Inferior Translation

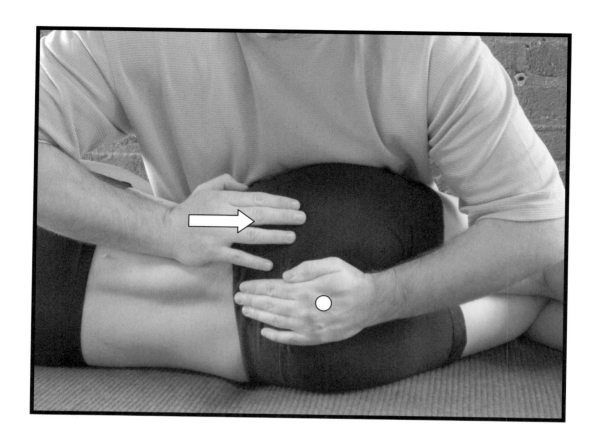

Technique described for the right SI joint

Patient: Left side lying with knees flexed

Therapist: Standing at the side of the bed. Stabilize the sacrum with the heel of your left hand. Palpate the iliac crest with the heel of your right hand.

Action: Apply an inferior translation force to the iliac crest. Note the end feel and reproduction of symptoms.

Stability Test
Pubic Symphysis Posterior Translation

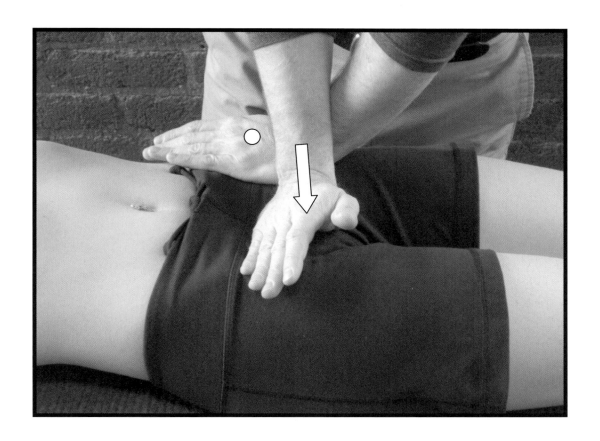

Technique described for the pubic symphysis

Patient: Supine lying

Therapist: Standing at the side of the bed. Stabilize the left innominate with your left hand. Palpate the right pubic tubercle with the ulnar border of your right hand.

Action: Apply a posterior translation force to the right pubic tubercle. Note the end feel and reproduction of symptoms. Switch your hands and apply a posterior translation force to the left pubic tubercle. Note the end feel and reproduction of symptoms.

Stability Test
Pubic Symphysis Inferior and Superior Translation

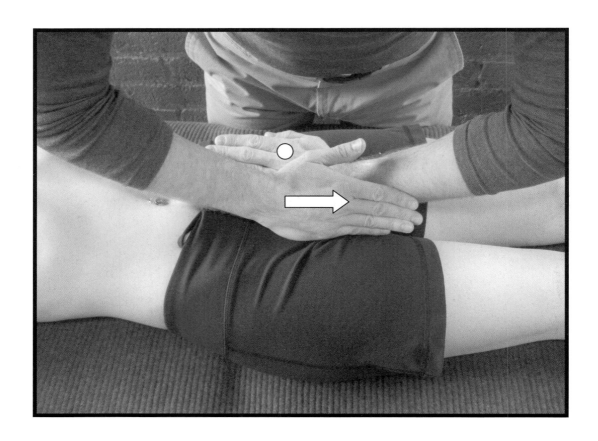

Technique described for the pubic symphysis

Patient: Supine lying

Therapist: Standing at the side of the bed. Stabilize the left pubic ramus with the ulnar border of your left hand. Palpate the right pubic tubercle with the ulnar border of your right hand.

Action: Apply an inferior translation force to the right pubic tubercle. Note the end feel and reproduction of symptoms.

For superior translation stabilize the left pubic ramus with your right hand and apply a superior translation force to the right pubic tubercle.

Ligament Stress Test
Anterior Gapping

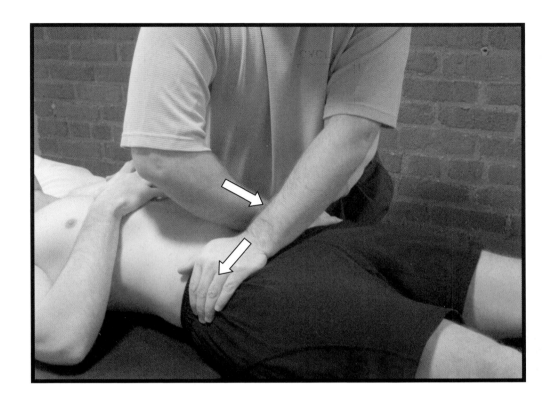

Patient: Supine lying

Therapist: Standing at the side of the bed. Place the heel of your right hand on the left ASIS. Place the heel of your left hand on the right ASIS.

Action: Apply a laterally directed force to both innominates. This will induce gapping at the anterior portion of the SI joints. Note the end feel and reproduction of symptoms.

Ligament Stress Test
Posterior Gapping

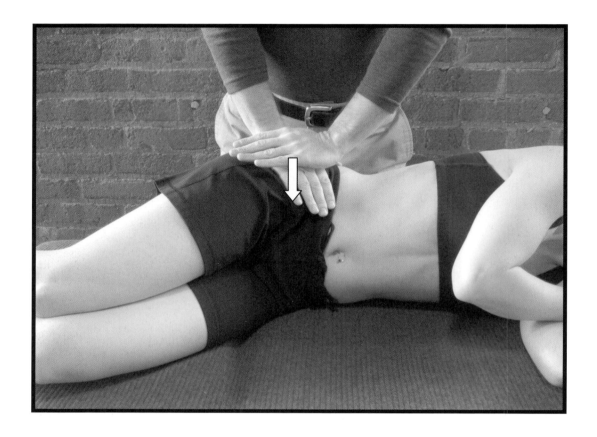

Patient: Left side lying with hips flexed

Therapist: Standing at the side of the bed. Place the heel of your right hand on the iliac crest and overlap with your left hand.

Action: Apply a compression force to the iliac crest. This will induce gapping at the posterior aspect of the SI joints. Note the end feel and reproduction of symptoms.

Ligament Stress Test
Long Dorsal SI Ligament

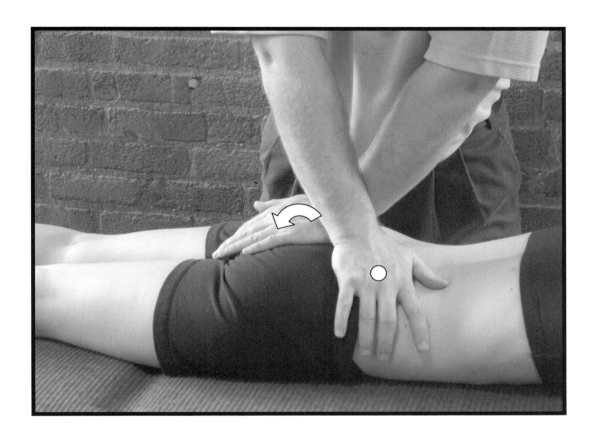

Technique described for the right SI joint

Patient: Prone lying

Therapist: Standing at the side of the bed. Stabilize the right PSIS with your right hand. Place the ulnar border of your left hand on the apex of the sacrum

Action: Passively counter-nutate the sacrum. This will stress the right long dorsal SI ligament. Note the end feel and reproduction of symptoms.

Ligament Stress Test
Sacrotuberous and Interosseous Ligament

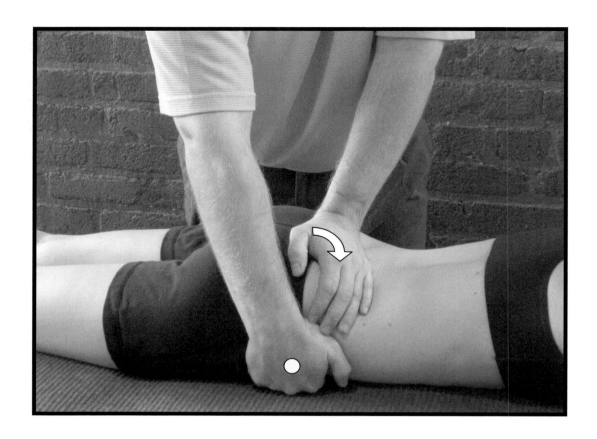

Technique described for the right SI joint

Patient: Prone lying

Therapist: Standing at the side of the bed. Stabilize the right ASIS with your right hand. Place the ulnar border of your left hand on the right sacral base.

Action: Passively nutate the sacrum. This will stress the right interosseous and sacrotuberous ligament. Note the end feel and reproduction of symptoms.

The Pelvis
Treatment Techniques

Treatment Technique
Innominate Anterior Rotation

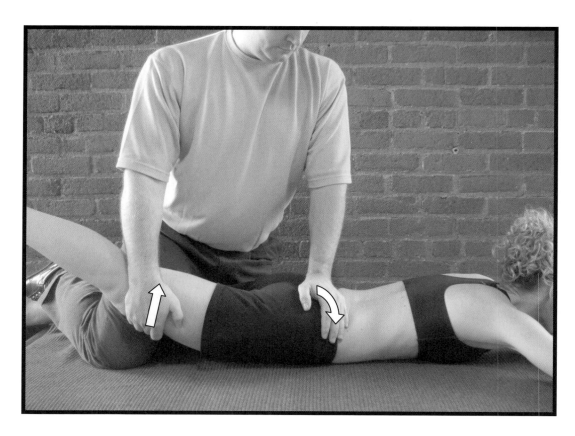

Technique described for the right SI joint

Indication: Articular restriction of anterior rotation

Patient: Prone lying at the edge of the bed

Therapist: Standing at the side of the bed. Place your right knee under the patient's right leg for support. Grasp the patient's distal femur with your right hand. Place the heel of your left hand over the right PSIS.

Action: Passively rotate the innominate to the restriction of motion. Apply an anterior directed force to the right innominate to facilitate anterior rotation. This technique can be graded from 1 to 4. Active mobilization can be utilized by instructing the patient to meet the therapists resistance at the motion barrier. Resist the direction which facilitates anterior rotation of the innominate. Hold the contraction for 5 seconds and then take up the new motion barrier. Repeat this process 3 times and then reassess your active and passive movement tests.

Treatment Technique
Innominate Posterior Rotation

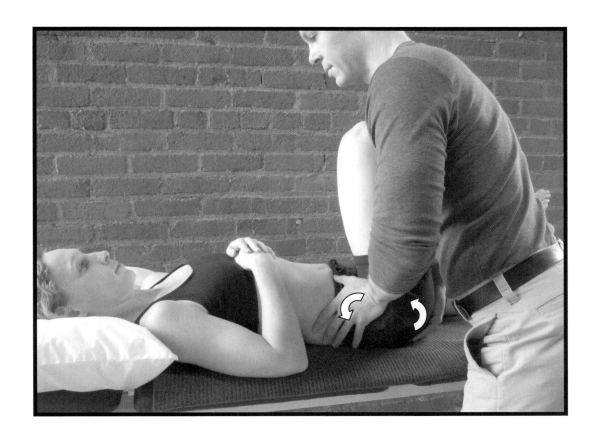

Technique described for the right SI joint

Indication: Articular restriction of posterior rotation

Patient: Supine lying

Therapist: Standing at the side of the bed. Flex the patient's hip to 90 degrees. Place your right hand under the right ischial tuberosity. Place your left hand over the right ASIS.

Action: Passively rotate the right innominate to the restriction of motion. Apply a posterior directed force to the ASIS and an anterior force to the right ischial tuberosity. This technique can be graded form 1 to 4.

Active mobilization can be utilized by instructing the patient to meet the therapists resistance at the motion barrier. Resist the direction which facilitates posterior rotation of the innominate. Hold the contraction for 5 seconds and then take up the new motion barrier. Repeat this process 3 times and then reassess your active and passive movement tests.

Treatment Technique
Unilateral Sacrum Nutation

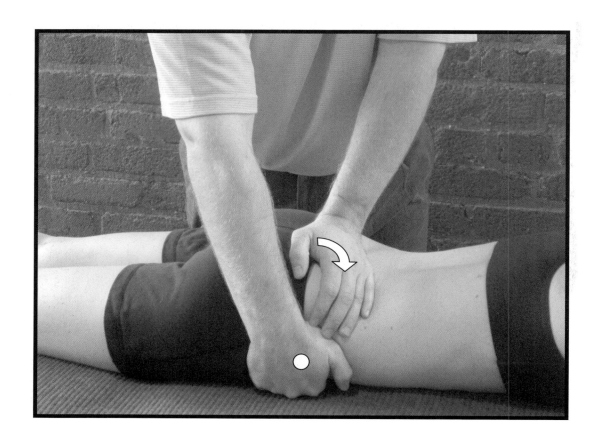

Technique described for the right SI joint

Indication: Unilateral articular restriction of sacral nutation

Patient: Prone lying

Therapist: Standing at the side of the bed. Stabilize the right ASIS with your right hand. Place the ulnar border of your left hand on the right sacral base.

Action: Mobilize the sacrum into nutation. This will induce an inferior-posterior glide of the sacrum on the innominate. This technique can be graded from 1 to 4.

Treatment Technique
Unilateral Sacrum Counternutation

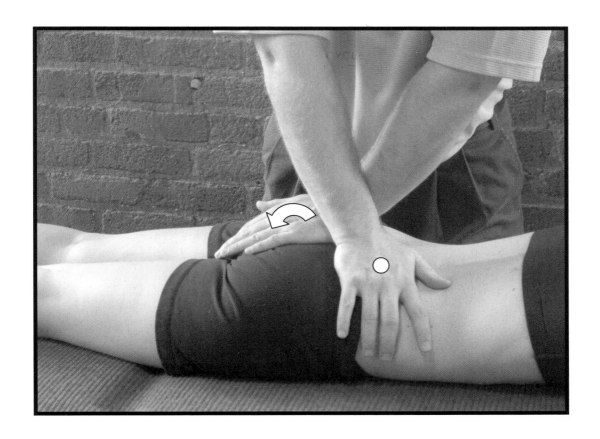

Technique described for the right SI joint

Indication: Unilateral restriction of sacral counternutation

Patient: Prone lying

Therapist: Standing at the side of the bed. Stabilize the right PSIS with your right hand. Place the ulnar border of your left hand on the apex of the sacrum

Action: Mobilize the sacrum into counternutation. This will induce an superior-anterior glide of the sacrum on the innominate. This technique can be graded from 1 to 4.

The Hip

The Hip
Active and Passive Movement Testing

Weight Bearing Range of Motion
Squat and Lunge

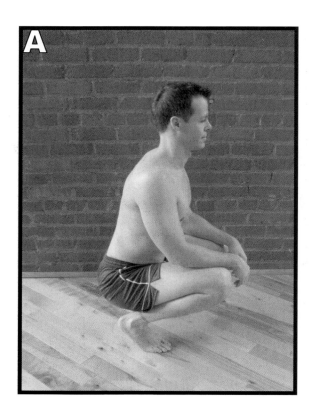

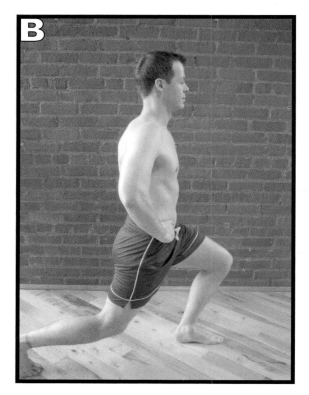

Technique described for the right hip joint

Patient: Standing without shoes

Therapist: Standing facing the patient

Action: Instruct the patient to perform a squat (A). Instruct the patient to perform a lunge (B). Observe the range of motion at the hip joint and note any reproduction of symptoms.

Weight Bearing Range of Motion
Single Leg Stance and Single Leg Squat

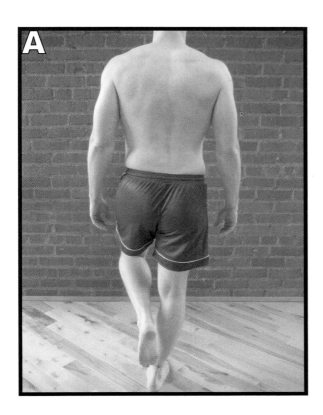 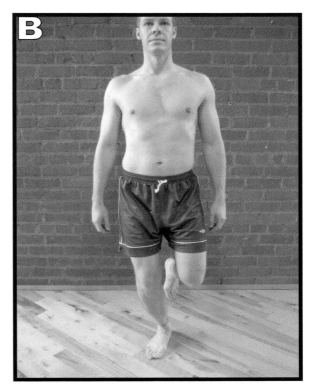

Technique described for the right hip joint

Patient: Standing without shoes

Therapist: Standing facing the patient

Action: Instruct the patient to stand on one leg (A). Instruct the patient to perform a single leg squat (B). Observe the range of motion at the hip joint and note any reproduction of symptoms.

Passive Range of Motion
Hip Flexion

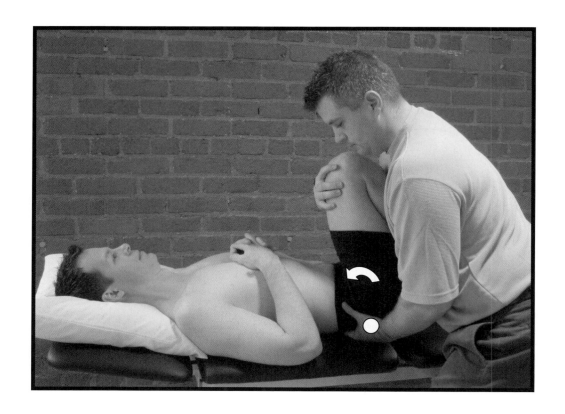

Technique described for the right hip joint

Patient: Supine lying

Therapist: Standing at the side of the bed. Stabilize the pelvis with your left hand. With the patient's knee flexed, grasp the distal femur with your right hand.

Action: Passively flex the patient's right hip. The end of the motion is reached when the pelvis begins to move. Note the range of motion, end feel and reproduction of symptoms.

Passive Range of Motion
Hip Extension

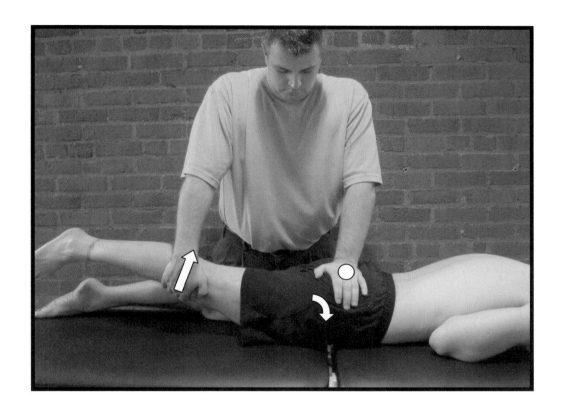

Technique described for the right hip

Patient: Prone lying

Therapist: Standing at the side of the bed. Stabilize the pelvis with your left hand. With the patient's knee, extended grasp the distal femur with your right hand.

Action: Passively extend the right hip. The end of the motion is reached when the pelvis begins to move. Note the range of motion, end feel and reproduction of symptoms.

Passive Range of Motion
Hip Abduction

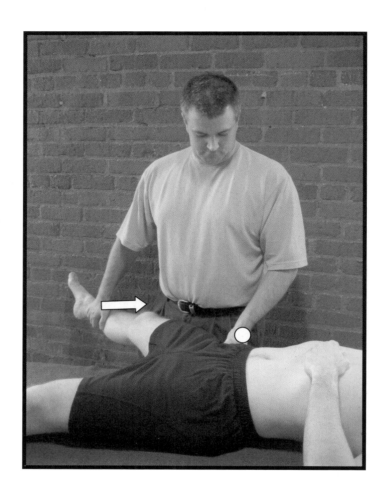

Technique described for the right hip

Patient: Supine lying

Therapist: Standing at the side of the bed. Stabilize the pelvis with your left hand. Grasp the distal tibia with your right hand.

Action: Passively abduct the patient's right hip. The end of the motion is reached when the pelvis begins to move. Note the range of motion, end feel and reproduction of symptoms.

Passive Range of Motion
Hip Adduction

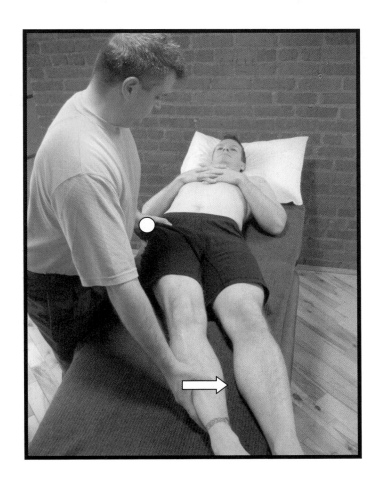

Technique described for the right hip

Patient: Supine lying with left leg abducted

Therapist: Standing at the side of the bed. Stabilize the pelvis with your left hand. Grasp the distal tibia with your right hand.

Action: Passively adduct the patient's right hip. The end of the motion is reached when the pelvis begins to move. Note the range of motion, end feel and reproduction of symptoms.

Passive Range of Motion
Internal and External Rotation In Flexion

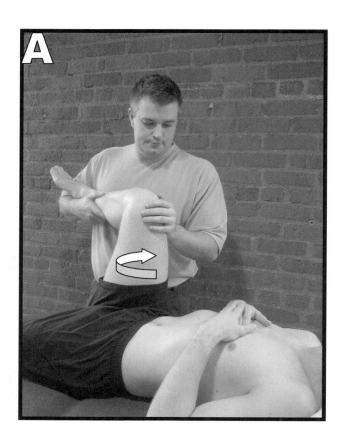
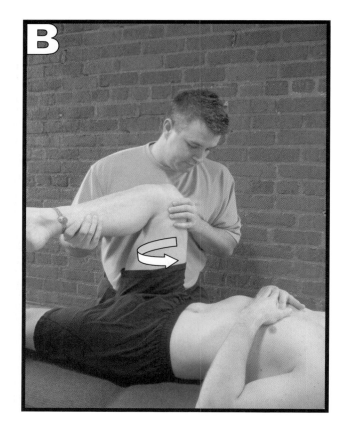

Technique described for the right hip

Patient: Supine lying with hip flexed

Therapist: Standing at the side of the bed. Place your left hand on the patient's right knee. Grasp the distal tibia with your right hand.

Action: Passively flex the patient's hip to 90 degrees and rotate the hip through internal (A) or external rotation (B). The end of the motion is reached when the pelvis begins to move. Note the range of motion, end feel and reproduction of symptoms.

Passive Range of Motion
Internal and External Rotation in Extension

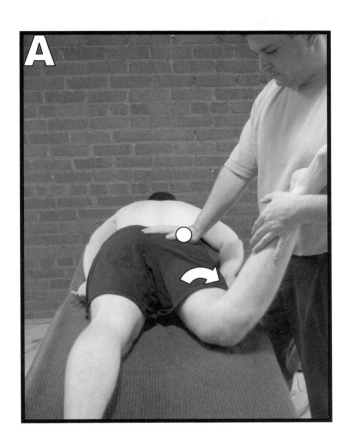

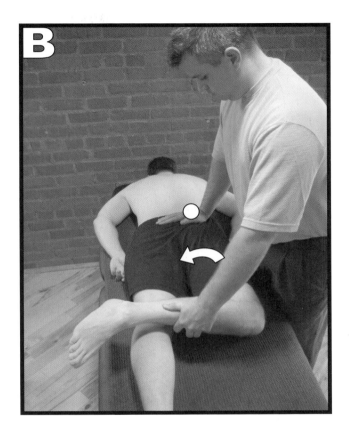

Technique described for the right hip

Patient: Prone lying with knee flexed

Therapist: Standing at the side of the bed. Stabilize the patient's pelvis with your right hand. Grasp the distal tibia with your left hand.

Action: Passively rotate the hip through internal rotation (A) or external rotation (B). The end of the motion is reached when the pelvis begins to move. Note the range of motion, end feel and reproduction of symptoms.

The hip can be biased into more extension by placing a rolled towel under the knee.

Passive Range of Motion
Combined Movement
Flexion-Adduction-Internal Rotation

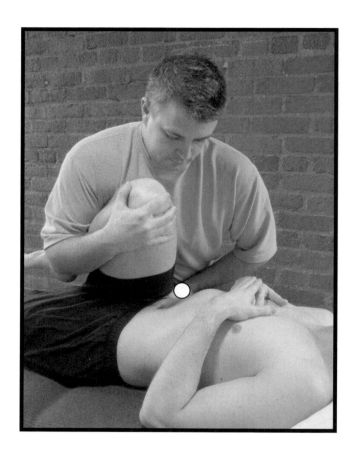

Technique described for the right hip

Patient: Supine lying with hip and knee flexed

Therapist: Standing at the side of the bed. Stabilize the pelvis with your left hand. Hold the patient's flexed knee between your right arm and thorax.

Action: Passively move the hip into flexion-adduction-internal rotation. The end of the motion is reached when the pelvis begins to move. Note the range of motion, end feel and reproduction of symptoms.

Passive Range of Motion
Combined Movement
Flexion-Abduction-External Rotation

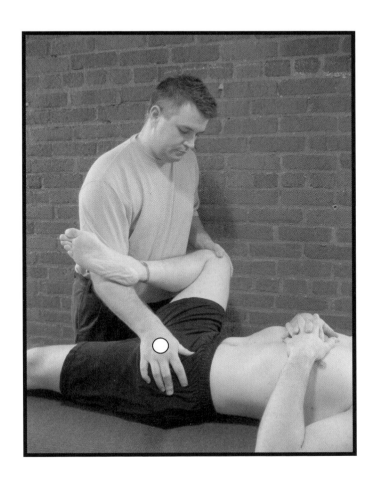

Technique described for the right hip

Patient: Supine lying hip and knee flexed

Therapist: Standing at the side of the bed. Stabilize the left side of the pelvis with your right hand. Grasp the distal femur with your left hand. You can control external rotation by placing the patient's foot on your right arm.

Action: Passively move the hip into flexion-abduction-external rotation. The end of the motion is reached when the pelvis begins to move. Note the range of motion, end feel and reproduction of symptoms.

Passive Range of Motion
Combined Movement
Extension-Adduction-Internal Rotation

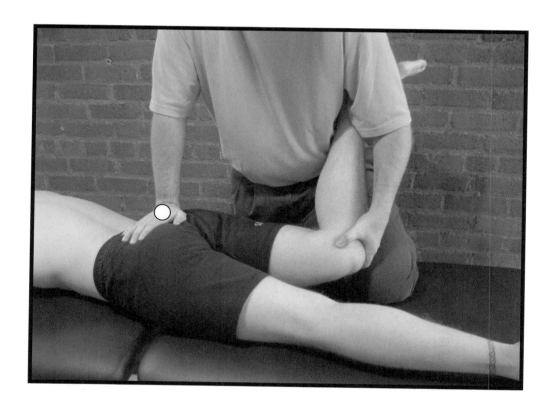

Technique described for the right hip

Patient: Prone lying with left leg abducted

Therapist: Standing at the side of the bed. Stabilize the pelvis with your right hand. With the patient's knee flexed, grasp the distal femur with your left hand.

Action: Passively move the patient's hip into extension-adduction-internal rotation. The end of the motion is reached when the pelvis begins to move. Note the range of motion, end feel and reproduction of symptoms.

Passive Range of Motion
Combined Movement
Extension-Abduction-External Rotation

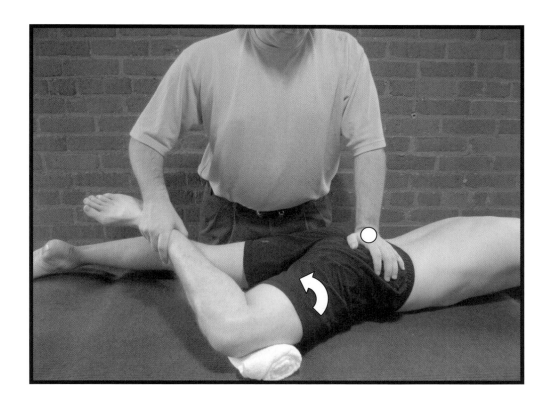

Technique described for the right hip

Patient: Prone lying with a rolled towel under right knee

Therapist: Standing at the side of the bed. Stabilize the pelvis with your left hand. With the patient's knee flexed, grasp the distal tibia with your right hand.

Action: Place the patient's hip in extension and abduction. Passively move the hip into external rotation. The end of the motion is reached when the pelvis begins to move. Note the range of motion, end feel and reproduction of symptoms.

Passive Accessory Motion
Anterior Glide

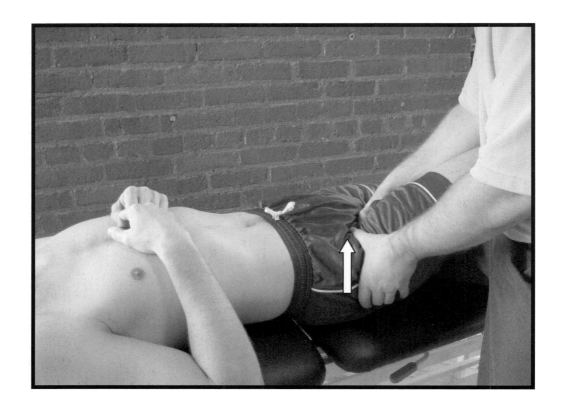

Technique described for the right hip

Patient: Supine lying with hip in 30 degrees of abduction and flexion

Therapist: Standing at the side of the bed. Support the patient's femur on your right thigh or a rolled towel. With both hands, grasp the right femur close to the joint line.

Action: Apply an anterior force to the femur. Note the range of motion, end feel and reproduction of symptoms.

Passive Accessory Motion
Posterior Glide

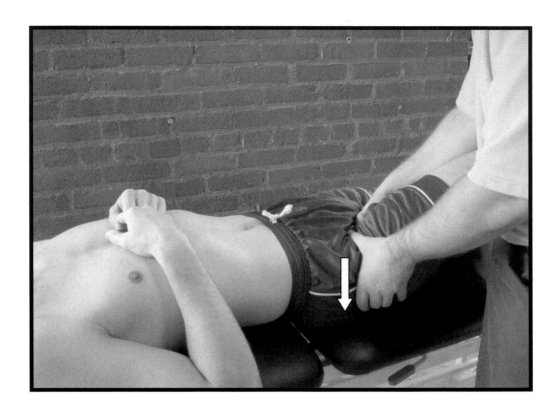

Technique described for the right hip

Patient: Supine lying with hip in 30 degrees of abduction and flexion

Therapist: Standing at the side of the bed. Support the patient's femur on your right thigh or a rolled towel. With both hands, grasp the right femur close to the joint line.

Action: Apply a posterior force to the femur. Note the range of motion, end feel and reproduction of symptoms.

Passive Accessory Motion
Inferior Glide

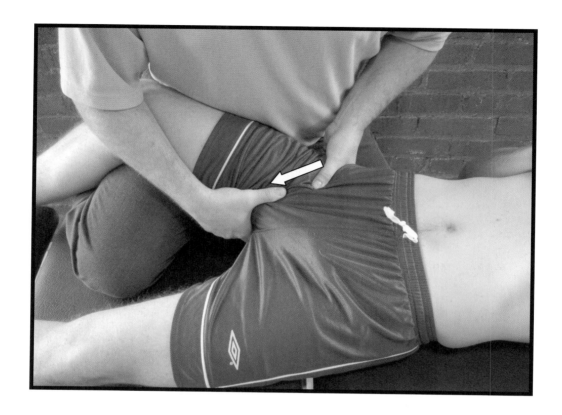

Technique described for the right hip

Patient: Supine lying with hip in 30 degrees of abduction and flexion

Therapist: Standing at the side of the bed. Support the patient's femur on your right thigh or a rolled towel. With both hands, grasp the right femur close to the joint line.

Action: Apply an inferior force to the femur. Note the range of motion, end feel and reproduction of symptoms.

Passive Accessory Motion
Superior Glide

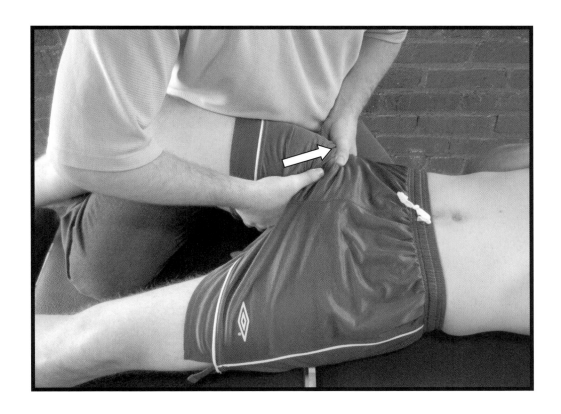

Technique described for the right hip

Patient: Supine lying with hip in 30 degrees of abduction and flexion

Therapist: Standing at the side of the bed. Support the patient's femur on your right thigh or a rolled towel. With both hands, grasp the right femur close to the joint line.

Action: Apply a superior force to the femur. Note the range of motion, end feel and reproduction of symptoms.

The Hip
Stability Testing

Stability Test
Compression and Traction

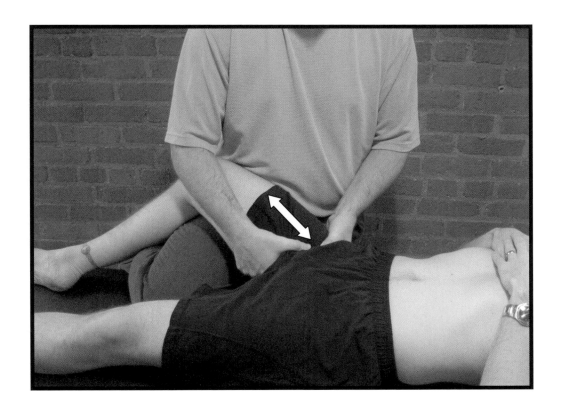

Technique described for the right hip

Patient: Supine lying with hip in 30 degrees of abduction and flexion

Therapist: Standing at the side of the bed. Support the patient's femur on your right thigh or a rolled towel. With both hands, grasp the right femur close to the joint line.

Action: Apply a compression or traction force to the femur. Note the end feel and reproduction of symptoms.

Stability Test
Anterior Translation

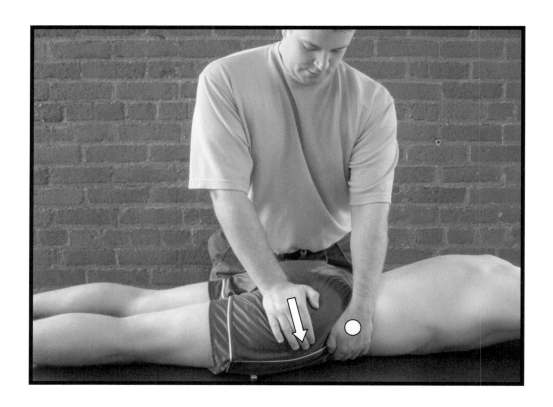

Technique described for the right hip

Patient: Prone lying

Therapist: Standing at the side of the bed. Stabilize the right innominate with your left hand. Place the right hand on the posterior aspect of the femoral head.

Action: Apply an anterior translation force to the femoral head. Note the end feel and reproduction of symptoms.

Stability Test
Posterior Translation

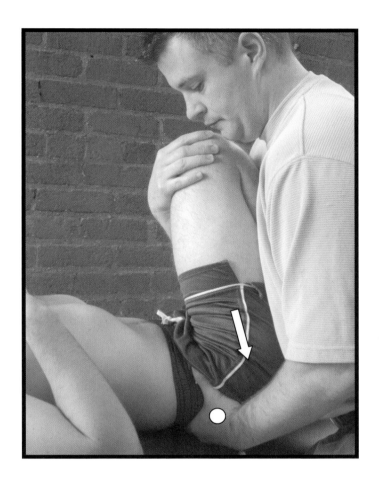

Technique described for the right hip

Patient: Supine lying with hip and knee flexed

Therapist: Standing at the side of the bed. Stabilize the right innominate with your left hand. Hold the patient's flexed knee between your right arm and thorax.

Action: Flex the patient's hip to 90 degrees and apply a posterior translation force to the femur. Note the end feel and reproduction of symptoms.

Stability Test
Inferior Translation

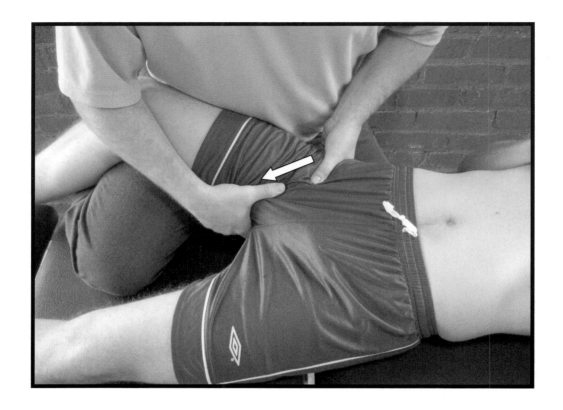

Technique described for the right hip

Patient: Supine lying with hip in 30 degrees of abduction and flexion

Therapist: Standing at the side of the bed. Support the patient's femur on your right thigh or a rolled towel. With both hands, grasp the right femur close to the joint line.

Action: Apply an inferior translation force to the femur. Note the end feel and reproduction of symptoms.

Stability Test
Superior Translation

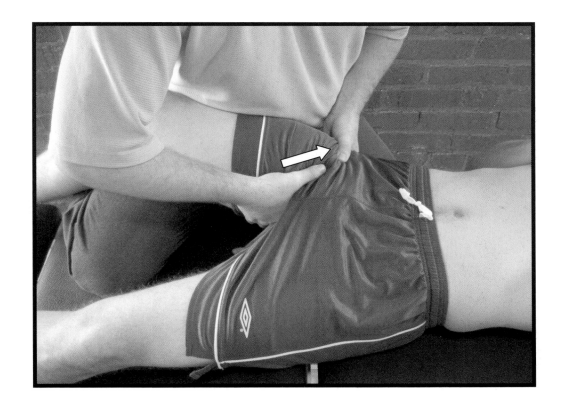

Technique described for the right hip

Patient: Supine lying with hip in 30 degrees of abduction and flexion

Therapist: Standing at the side of the bed. Support the patient's femur on your right thigh or a rolled towel. With both hands, grasp the right femur close to the joint line.

Action: Apply a superior translation force to the femur. Note the end feel and reproduction of symptoms.

Ligament Stress Test
Torque Test (Lee 2005)

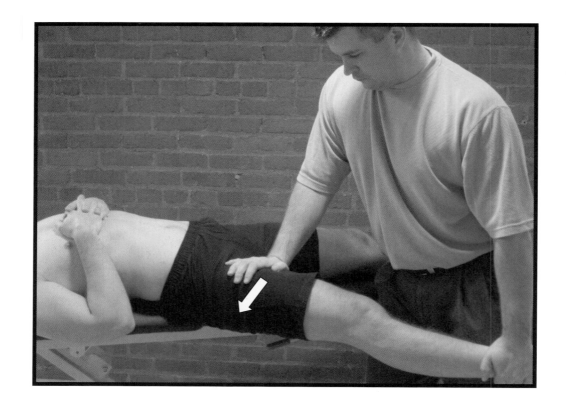

Technique described for the right hip. This position will stress all capsular ligaments of the hip joint.

Patient: Supine lying at edge of the bed

Therapist: Standing between the patient's leg and the bed. Grasp the distal tibia and fibula with your left hand. Place the right hand on the medial aspect of the femur close to the joint line.

Action: Move the patient's hip into extension and internal rotation. Apply a posterior-lateral force to the femur to distract the hip joint. Note the end feel and reproduction of symptoms.

Ligament Stress Test
Inferior Band of the Iliofemoral Ligament

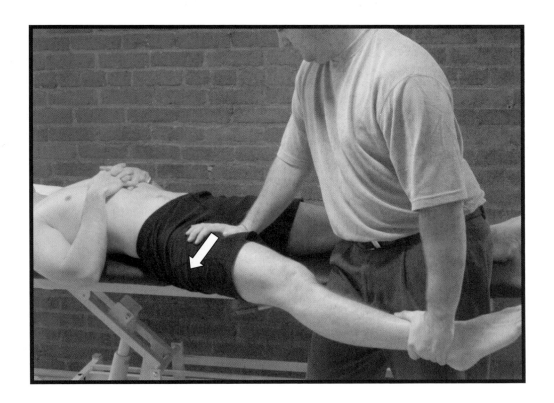

Technique described for the right hip

Patient: Supine lying at edge of the bed

Therapist: Standing between the patient's leg and the bed. Grasp the distal tibia and fibula with your left hand. Place the right hand on the medial aspect of the femur close to the joint line.

Action: Move the patient's hip into extension, abduction and internal rotation. Apply a posterior-lateral force to the femur to distract the hip joint. Note the end feel and reproduction of symptoms.

Ligament Stress Test
Iliotrochanteric Band of the Iliofemoral Ligament

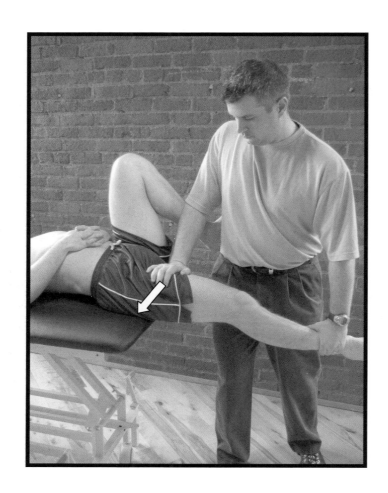

Technique described for the right hip

Patient: Supine lying with the left hip flexed and foot resting on the therapist's thorax

Therapist: Standing at the end of the bed. Grasp the distal tibia and fibula with your left hand. Place your right hand over the anterior-medial aspect of the femur close to the joint line.

Action: Move the patient's hip into extension, adduction and external rotation. Apply a lateral force to the femur to distract the hip joint. Note the end feel and reproduction of symptoms.

Ligament Stress Test
Pubofemoral Ligament

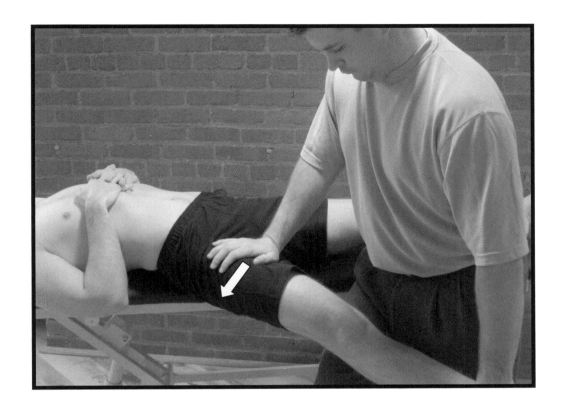

Technique described for the right hip

Patient: Supine lying at edge of the bed

Therapist: Standing between the patient's leg and the bed. Grasp the distal tibia and fibula with your left hand. Place the right hand on the medial aspect of the femur close to the joint line.

Action: Move the patient's hip into extension, abduction and external rotation. Apply a posterior-lateral force to the femur to distract the hip joint. Note the end feel and reproduction of symptoms.

Ligament Stress Test
Ischiofemoral Ligament

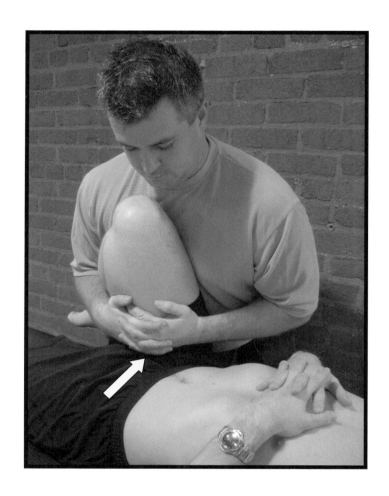

Technique described for the right hip

Patient: Supine lying with hip and knee flexed

Therapist: Standing at the side of the bed. Place both hands on the patient's femur close to the joint line.

Action: Move the patient's hip into flexion-adduction-internal rotation. Apply a lateral force to the femur. Note the end feel and reproduction of symptoms.

The Hip
Treatment Techniques

Passive Physiological Mobilization

Passive Accessory Mobilization

Treatment Technique
Passive Physiological Mobilization
Flexion

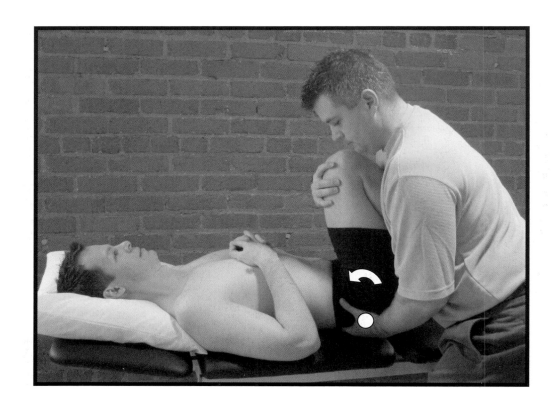

Technique described for the right hip

Indication: Restriction of hip flexion

Patient: Supine lying

Therapist: Stabilize the pelvis with your left hand. With the patient's knee flexed, grasp the distal femur with your right hand.

Action: Mobilize the hip into flexion. This technique can be graded from 1 to 4.

Treatment Technique
Passive Physiological Mobilization
Extension

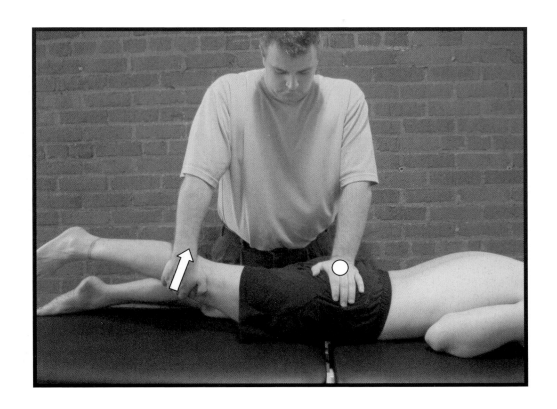

Technique described for the right hip

Indication: Restriction of hip extension

Patient: Prone lying with knee extended

Therapist: Stabilize the pelvis with your left hand. Grasp the distal femur with your right hand.

Action: Mobilize the hip into extension. This technique can be graded from 1 to 4.

Treatment Technique
Passive Physiological Mobilization
Abduction

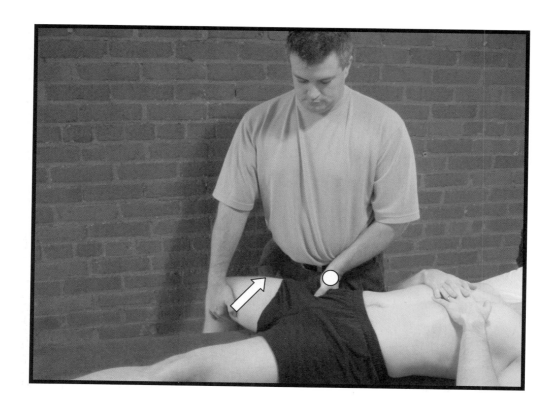

Technique described for the right hip

Indication: Restriction of hip abduction

Patient: Supine lying at edge of the bed

Therapist: Grasp the distal femur with your right hand. Stabilize the pelvis with your left hand.

Action: Mobilize the hip into abduction. This technique can be graded from 1 to 4.

Treatment Technique
Passive Physiological Mobilization
Adduction

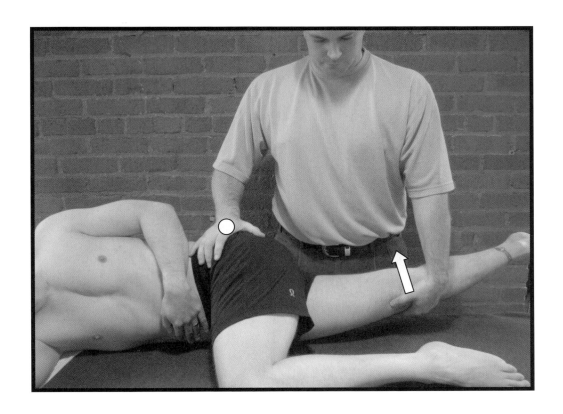

Technique described for the right hip

Indication: Restriction of hip adduction

Patient: Right side lying with left hip and knee flexed resting on the bed

Therapist: Standing at the side of the bed. Stabilize the pelvis with your right hand. Grasp the distal femur with your left hand.

Action: Mobilize the hip into adduction. This technique can be graded from 1 to 4.

Treatment Technique
Passive Physiological Mobilization
Internal Rotation and External Rotation in Flexion

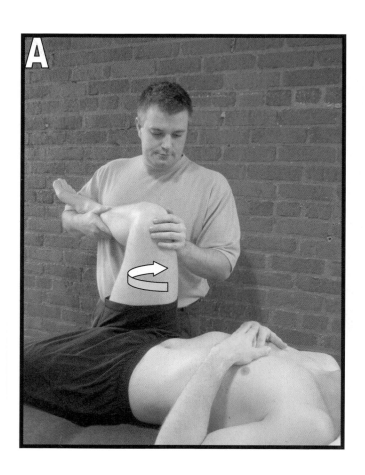

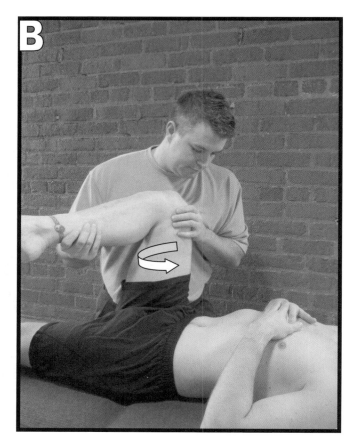

Technique described for the right hip

Indication: Restriction of internal rotation or external rotation in hip flexion

Patient: Supine lying with hip and knee flexed

Therapist: Place the left hand on the patient's right knee. Grasp the distal tibia with your right hand.

Action: Mobilize the hip into internal rotation (A) or external rotation (B). This technique can be graded from 1 to 4.

Treatment Technique
Passive Physiological Mobilization
Internal Rotation In Extension

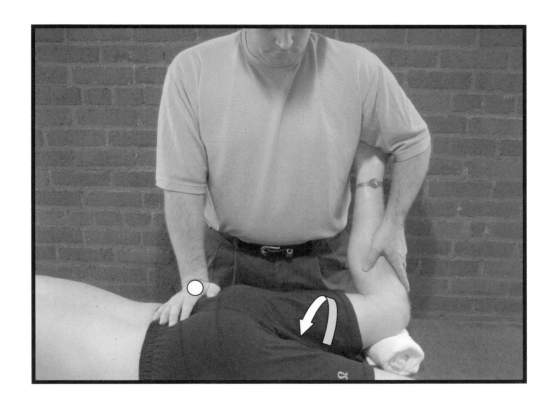

Technique described for the right hip

Indication: Restriction of internal rotation in extension

Patient: Prone lying with knee flexed and a rolled towel under the knee

Therapist: Stabilize the patient's pelvis with your right hand. Grasp the proximal tibia with your left hand.

Action: Mobilize the hip into internal rotation. This technique can be graded form 1 to 4.

Treatment Technique
Passive Physiological Mobilization
External Rotation In Extension

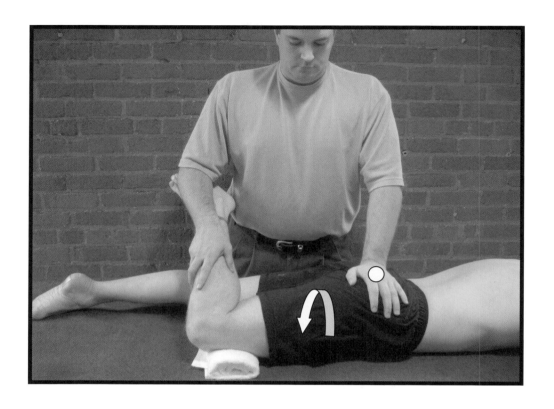

Technique described for the right hip

Indication: Restriction of external rotation in extension

Patient: Prone lying with knee flexed and rolled towel under knee

Therapist: Stabilize the patient's pelvis with your left hand. Grasp the tibia with your right hand.

Action: Mobilize the hip into external rotation. This technique can be graded form 1 to 4.

Treatment Technique
Passive Physiological Mobilization
Combined Flexion-Adduction-Internal Rotation

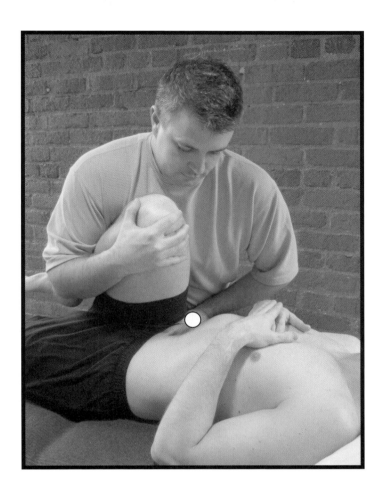

Technique described for the right hip

Indication: Restriction of flexion-adduction-internal rotation

Patient: Supine lying hip and knee flexed

Therapist: Standing at the side of the bed. Stabilize the pelvis with your left hand. Hold the patient's flexed knee between your right arm and thorax.

Action: Mobilize the hip into flexion-adduction-internal rotation. This technique can be graded from 1 to 4.

Treatment Technique
Passive Physiological Mobilization
Combined Flexion-Abduction-External Rotation

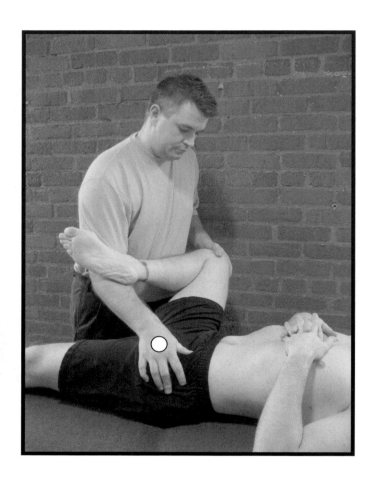

Technique described for the right hip

Indication: Restriction of flexion-abduction-external rotation

Patient: Supine lying hip and knee flexed

Therapist: Standing at the side of the bed. Stabilize the left side of the pelvis with your right hand. Grasp the distal femur with your left hand. You can control external rotation by placing the patient's foot on your right arm.

Action: Mobilize the hip into flexion-abduction-external rotation. This technique can be graded from 1 to 4.

Treatment Technique
Passive Physiological Mobilization
Combined Extension-Abduction-External Rotation

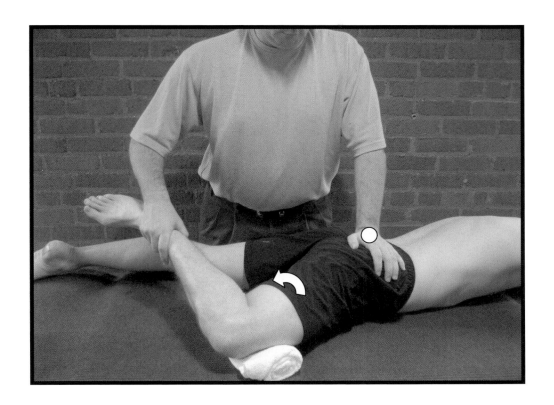

Technique described for the right hip

Indication: Restriction of extension-abduction-external rotation

Patient: Prone lying with hip abducted and a rolled towel under flexed right knee

Therapist: Standing at the side of the bed. Stabilize the right side of the pelvis with your left hand. Grasp the distal tibia with your right hand.

Action: Mobilize the hip into external rotation. This technique can be graded from 1 to 4.

Treatment Technique
Passive Physiological Mobilization
Combined Extension-Adduction-Internal Rotation

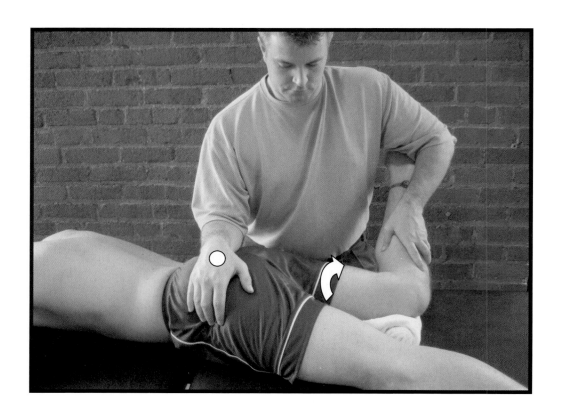

Technique described for the right hip

Indication: Restriction of extension-adduction-internal rotation

Patient: Prone lying with hip adducted and rolled towel under flexed right knee

Therapist: Standing at the side of the bed. Stabilize the pelvis with your right forearm. Grasp the proximal tibia with your left hand.

Action: Mobilize the hip into internal rotation. This technique can be graded from 1 to 4.

Treatment Technique
Distraction – Loose Pack Position
(With A Belt)

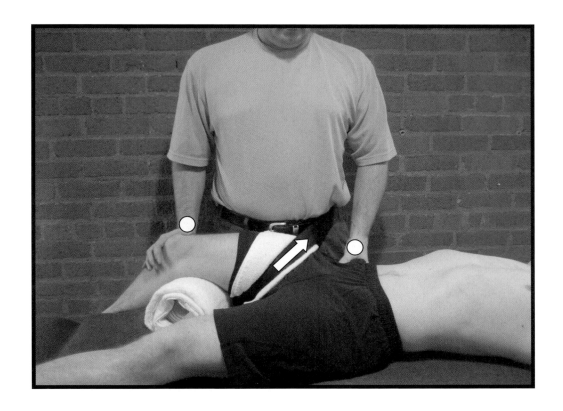

Technique described for the right hip

Indication: Articular restriction of the hip joint

Patient: Supine lying with hip in 30 degrees of abduction and flexion

Therapist: Standing at the side of the bed. Support the patient's femur with a rolled towel. Wrap a mobilization belt around the patient's femur close to the joint line. Place a towel between the patient's thigh and the belt for comfort. Wrap the belt around your pelvis. Stabilize the distal femur with your right hand and the pelvis with your left hand.

Action: Apply a distraction force to the hip by shifting your weight backward. This technique can be graded from 1 to 4.

Treatment Technique
Distraction in Flexion
(With a Belt)

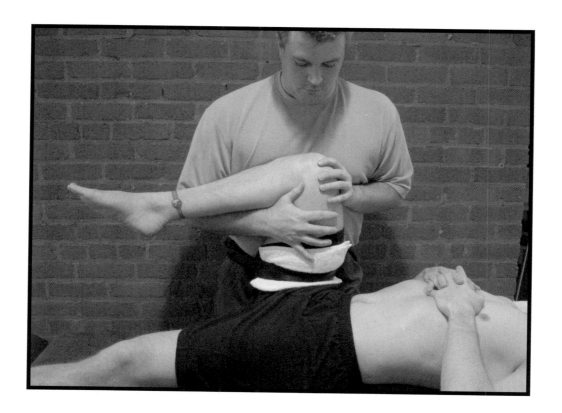

Technique described for the right hip

Indication: Articular restriction of the hip joint in a flexed position

Patient: Supine lying with hip and knee flexed

Therapist: Standing at the side of the bed. Wrap a mobilization belt around the patient's femur close to the joint line. Place a towel between the patient's thigh and the belt for comfort. Wrap the belt around your pelvis. Hold the distal femur against your thorax with both hands.

Action: Apply a distraction force to the hip by shifting your weight backward. This technique can be graded from 1 to 4. Combinations of abduction / adduction, and internal / external rotation can be used depending on the movement restriction.

Treatment Technique
Distraction in Extension
(With a Belt)

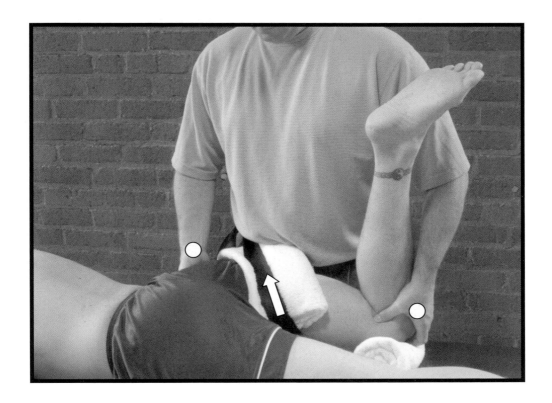

Technique described for the right hip

Indication: Articular restriction of the hip joint in extension

Patient: Prone lying with rolled towel under flexed right knee

Therapist: Standing at the side of the bed. Wrap a mobilization belt around the patient's femur close to the joint line. Place a towel between the patient's thigh and the belt for comfort. Wrap the belt around your pelvis. Stabilize the patient's pelvis with your right hand. Grasp the distal femur with your left hand.

Action: Apply a distraction force to the hip by shifting your weight backward. This technique can be graded from 1 to 4. Combinations of abduction / adduction, and internal / external rotation can be used depending on the movement restriction.

Treatment Technique
Anterior Glide

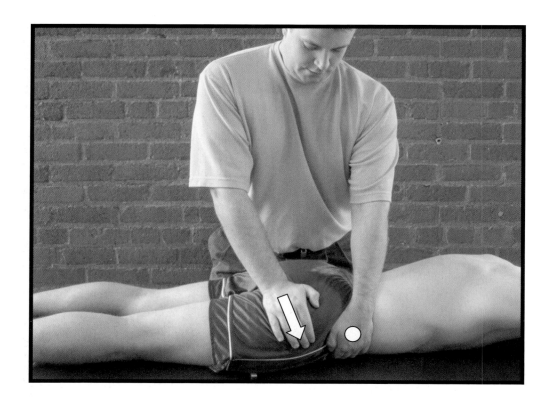

Technique described for the right hip

Indication: Articular restriction of extension and / or external rotation

Patient: Prone lying

Therapist: Standing at the side of the bed. Stabilize the right innominate with your left hand. Place the right hand on the posterior aspect of the femoral head.

Action: Apply an anterior glide to the femoral head. This technique can be graded from 1 to 4.

Treatment Technique
Posterior Glide

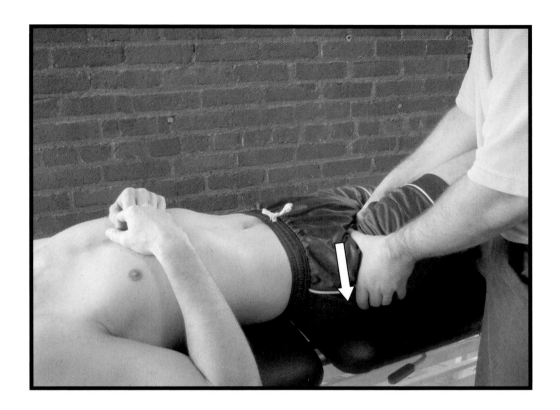

Technique described for the right hip

Indication: Articular restriction of flexion and/or internal rotation

Patient: Supine lying with hip in 30 degrees of abduction and flexion

Therapist: Standing at the side of the bed. Support the patient's femur on your right thigh or a rolled towel. With both hands, grasp the right femur close to the joint line.

Action: Apply a posterior glide to the femur. This technique can be graded from 1 to 4.

Treatment Technique
Inferior Glide

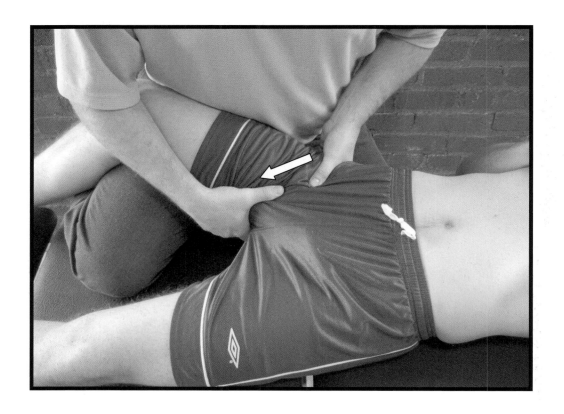

Technique described for the right hip

Indication: Articular restriction of abduction

Patient: Supine lying with hip in 30 degrees of abduction and flexion

Therapist: Standing at the side of the bed. Support the patient's femur on your right thigh or a rolled towel. With both hands, grasp the right femur close to the joint line.

Action: Apply an inferior glide to the femur. This technique can be graded from 1 to 4.

Treatment Technique
Superior Glide

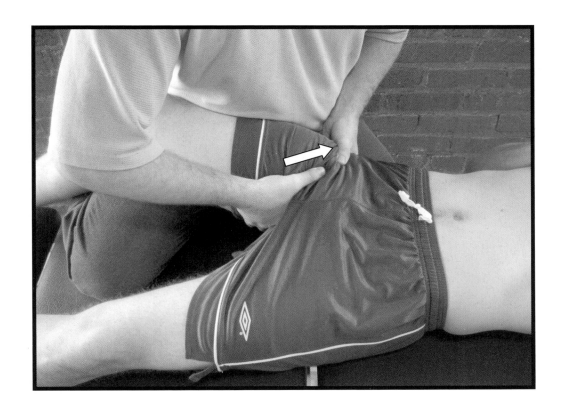

Technique described for the right hip

Indication: Articular restriction of adduction

Patient: Supine lying with hip in 30 degrees of abduction and flexion

Therapist: Standing at the side of the bed. Support the patient's femur on your right thigh or a rolled towel. With both hands, grasp the right femur close to the joint line.

Action: Apply a superior glide to the femur. This technique can be graded from 1 to 4.

The Knee

The Knee
Active and Passive Movement Testing

Weight Bearing Range of Motion
Squat

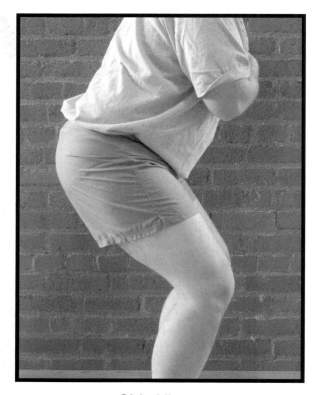

Side View

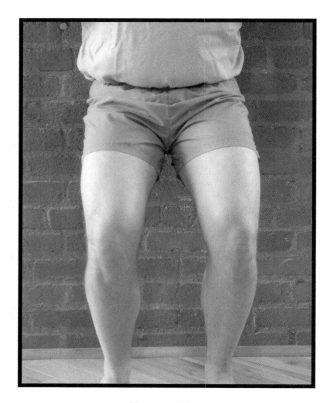

Front View

Technique described for the right knee

Patient: Standing without shoes

Therapist: Seated or kneeling

Action: Instruct the patient to perform a squat. Observe the range of motion at the tibio-femoral, superior tibio-fibular and patello-femoral joints and note any reproduction of symptoms.

Weight Bearing Range of Motion
Single Leg Squat

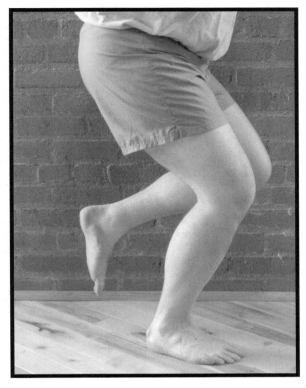

Side View

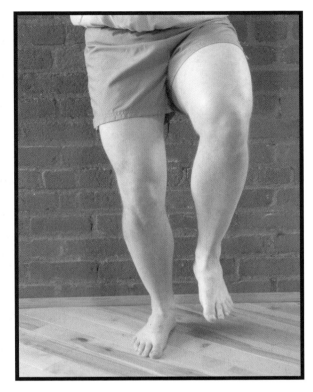

Front View

Technique described for the right knee

Patient: Standing without shoes

Therapist: Seated or kneeling

Action: Instruct the patient to perform a single leg squat. Observe the range of motion at the tibio-femoral, superior tibio-fibular and patello-femoral joints and note any reproduction of symptoms.

Weight Bearing Range of Motion
Body Twist and Heel Raise

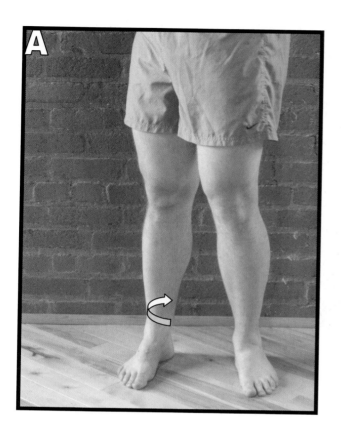

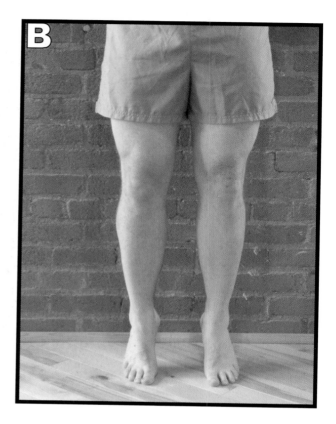

Technique described for the right knee

Patient: Standing without shoes

Therapist: Seated or kneeling

Action: Instruct the patient to twist their body to the right (A). Instruct the patient to rise up on their toes (B). Observe the range of motion at the tibio-femoral, superior tibio-fibular and patello-femoral joints and note any reproduction of symptoms. Repeat for left body twist.

Active Range of Motion
Extension (Open Kinetic Chain)

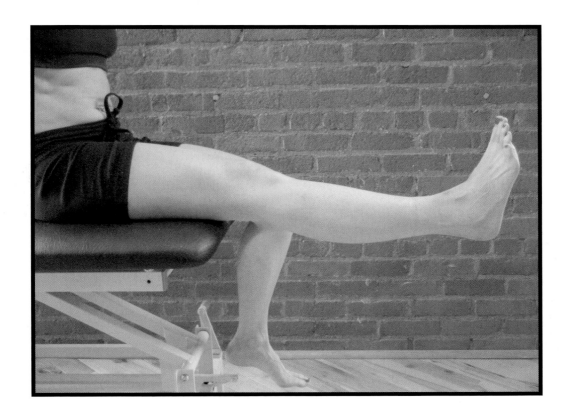

Technique described for right knee

Patient: Seated at the edge of the bed knee flexed

Therapist: Seated in front of the patient

Action: Instruct the patient to actively extend the knee joint. Observe the range of motion at the tibio-femoral and patello-femoral joints and note any reproduction of symptoms.

Active Range of Motion
Internal and External Rotation (Open Kinetic Chain)

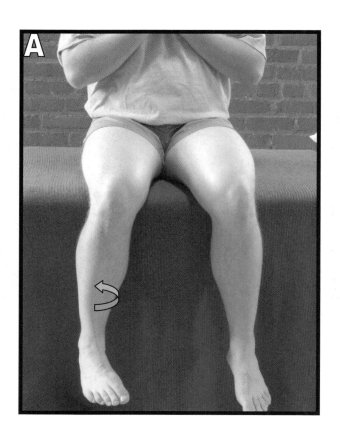 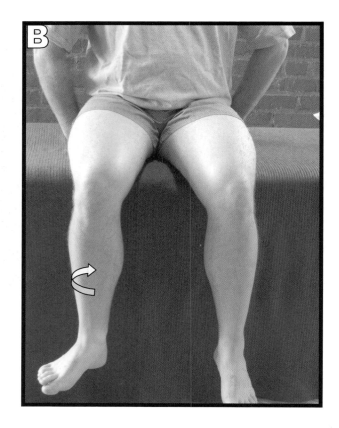

Technique described for right knee

Patient: Seated at the edge of the bed

Therapist: Seated in front of the patient

Action: Instruct the patient to actively rotate the tibia medially (A) and laterally (B). Make sure that the hip joint remains in neutral. Observe the range of motion at the tibio-femoral and superior tibio-fibular joints and note any reproduction of symptoms.

Passive Range of Motion
Flexion and Extension

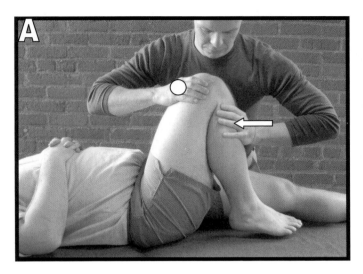

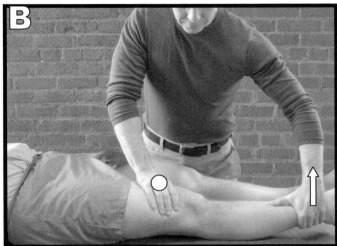

Technique described for right knee

Patient: Supine lying

Therapist: Standing at the side of the patient. Stabilize the femur with your right hand while grasping the proximal tibia with your left hand.

Action: Passively flex the tibo-femoral joint (A). For extension (B), you may want to grasp the distal aspect of the tibia with your left hand to get better leverage. Note the range of motion, end feel and reproduction of symptoms.

Passive Range of Motion
Internal Rotation & External Rotation

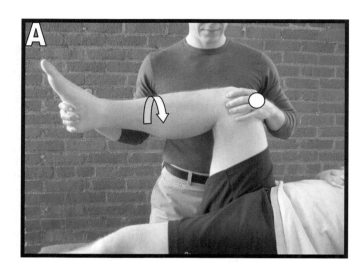 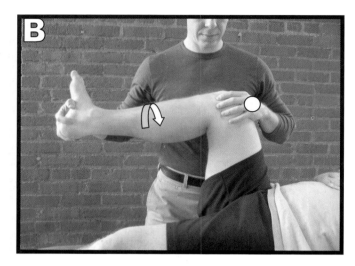

Technique described for right knee

Patient: Supine with hip and knee flexed to 90 degrees

Therapist: Standing at the side of the patient. With the left hand, stabilize the distal femur while palpating the tibio-femoral joint line. Grasp the distal tibia (or calcaneus) with the right hand.

Action: Passively rotate the tibia medially (A) and laterally (B). Note the range of motion, end feel and reproduction of symptoms.

Passive Range of Motion
Combined Movements
Flexion / Abduction and Flexion / Adduction

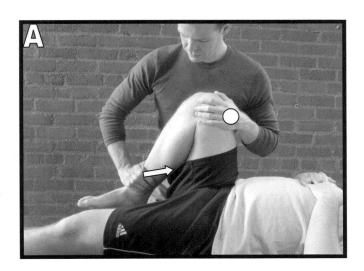 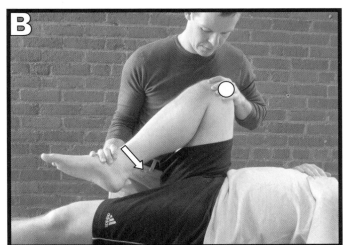

Technique described for right knee

Patient: Supine with hip flexed to 90 degrees

Therapist: Standing at the side of the patient. With the left hand, stabilize the distal femur while palpating the tibio-femoral joint line. Grasp the distal tibia with the right hand.

Action: Passively flex and abduct the tibia (A) then flex and adduct the tibia (B). Each of these movements can be further biased into medial and lateral rotation. Note the range of motion, end feel and reproduction of symptoms.

Passive Range of Motion
Combined Movements
Extension / Abduction and Extension / Adduction

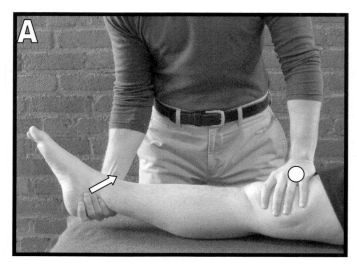 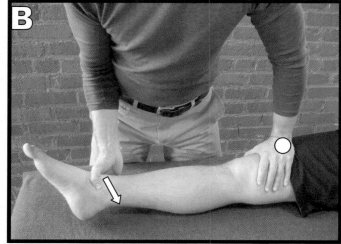

Technique described for right knee

Patient: Supine

Therapist: Standing at the side of the patient. With the left hand, stabilize the distal femur while palpating the tibio-femoral joint line. Grasp the distal tibia with the right hand.

Action: Passively extend and abduct the tibia (A) then extend and adduct the tibia (B). Each of these movements can be further biased into medial and lateral rotation. Note the range of motion, end feel and reproduction of symptoms.

Passive Accessory Motion
Tibio-Femoral Anterior Glide

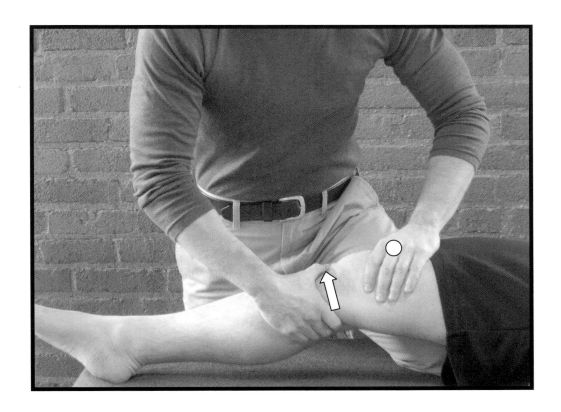

Technique described for right tibio-femoral joint

Patient: Supine with knee flexed to 30 degrees

Therapist: Standing at the side of the bed. Support the patient's thigh with your left leg or a rolled towel. Stabilize the distal femur with your left hand. Grasp the proximal tibia with your right hand.

Action: Apply an anterior force to the tibia. Note the range of motion, end feel and reproduction of symptoms. This glide can also be assessed at the restriction of extension.

Passive Accessory Motion
Tibio-Femoral Posterior Glide

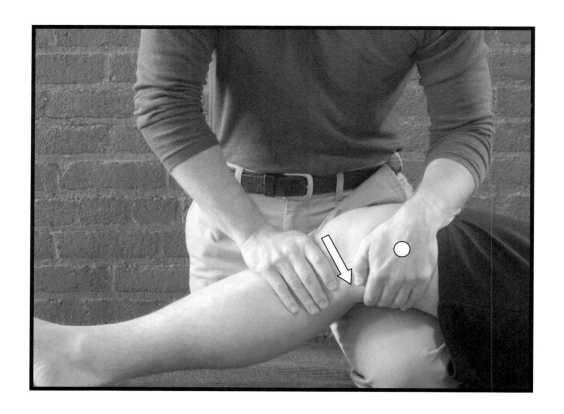

Technique described for right tibio-femoral joint

Patient: Supine with knee flexed to 30 degrees

Therapist: Standing at the side of the bed. Support the patient's thigh with your left leg or a rolled towel. Stabilize the distal femur with your left hand. Grasp the proximal tibia with your right hand.

Action: Apply a posterior force to the tibia. Note the range of motion, end feel and reproduction of symptoms. This glide can also be assessed at the restriction of flexion.

Passive Accessory Motion
Tibio-Femoral Medial Glide

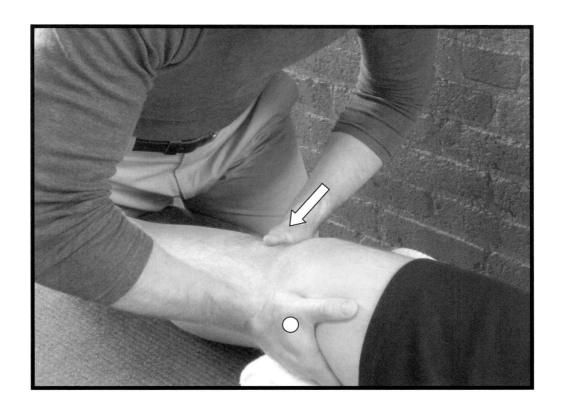

Technique described for the right tibio-femoral joint

Patient: Supine with a rolled towel under knee

Therapist: Standing at the side of the bed. Stabilize the medial aspect of the distal femur with your right hand. Grasp the lateral aspect of the proximal tibia with your left hand.

Action: Apply a medial force to the tibia. Note the range of motion, end feel and reproduction of symptoms.

Passive Accessory Motion
Tibio-Femoral Lateral Glide

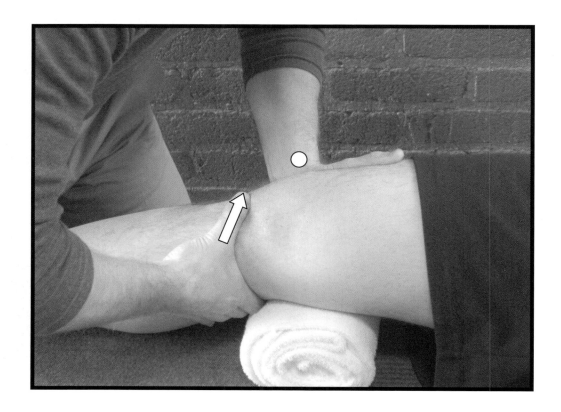

Technique described for the right tibio-femoral joint

Patient: Supine with a rolled towel under knee

Therapist: Standing at the side of the bed. Stabilize the lateral aspect of the distal femur with your left hand. Grasp the medial aspect of the proximal tibia with your right hand.

Action: Apply a lateral force to the tibia. Note the range of motion, end feel and reproduction of symptoms.

Passive Accessory Motion
Patello-Femoral Joint
Superior / Inferior / Medial / Lateral Glide

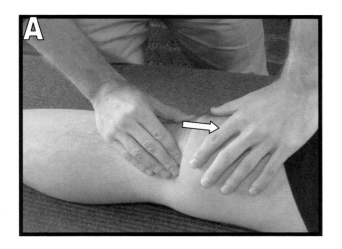

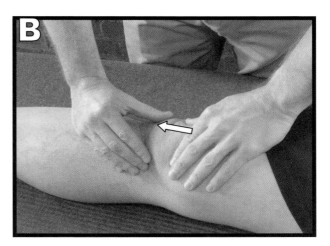

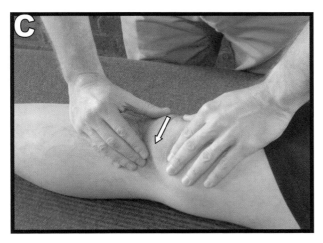

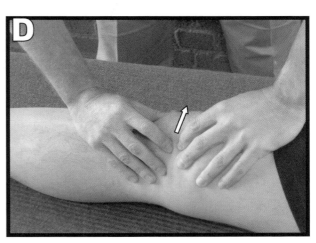

Technique described for the right patello-femoral joint

Patient: Supine with knee extended

Therapist: Standing at the side of the bed. Grasp the distal aspect of the patella with your right thumb and index finger. Grasp the proximal aspect of the patella with your left thumb and index finger.

Action: Apply a superior force to the patella with your right hand while controlling the patella with your left hand (A). Note the range of motion, end feel and reproduction of symptoms. Repeat for an inferior glide (B), medial glide (C), and lateral glide (D).

Passive Accessory Motion
Superior Tibio-Fibular Joint
Anterior Glide

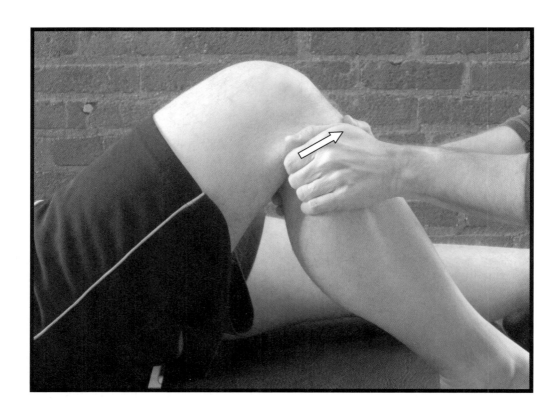

Technique described for the right superior tibio-fibular joint

Patient: Supine with knee flexed to 90 degrees

Therapist: Standing at the side of the bed facing the patient. Stabilize the proximal tibia with your right hand. Grasp the head of the fibula between the thenar eminence and index and middle fingers of your left hand.

Action: Apply an anterior force to the head of the fibula. Note the range of motion, end feel and reproduction of symptoms.

Passive Accessory Motion
Superior Tibio-Fibular Joint
Posterior Glide

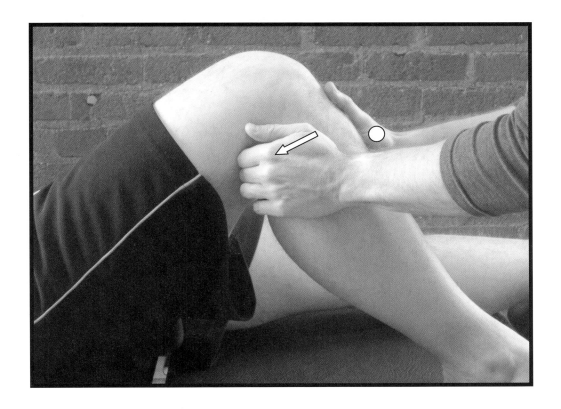

Technique described for the right superior tibio-fibular joint

Patient: Supine with knee flexed to 90 degrees

Therapist: Standing at the side of the bed facing the patient. Stabilize the proximal tibia with your right hand. Grasp the head of the fibula between the thenar eminence and index and middle fingers of your left hand.

Action: Apply a posterior force to the head of the fibula. Note the range of motion, end feel and reproduction of symptoms.

The Knee
Stability Tests

Stability Test
Tibio-Femoral Joint
Compression and Traction

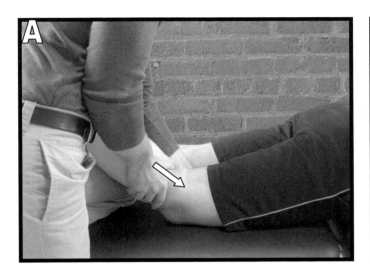 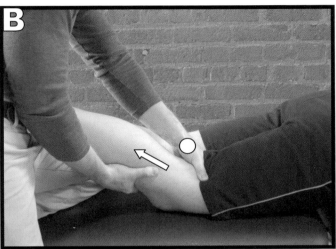

Technique described for the right tibio-femoral joint

Patient: Prone with knee flexed to 30 degrees

Therapist: Standing at the side of the bed. Stabilize the distal femur with your left hand. Grasp the proximal tibia with your right hand.

Action: Apply a compressive force along the line of the tibia (A). Repeat using a traction force along the line of the tibia (B). Note the end feel and reproduction of symptoms.

Stability Test
Tibio-Femoral Joint
Anterior Drawer

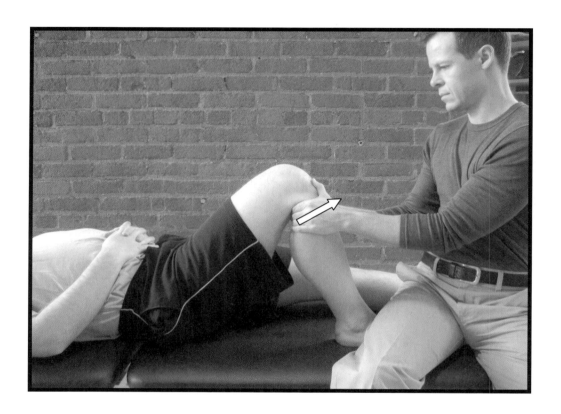

Technique described for the right tibio-femoral joint

Patient: Supine with knee flexed to 90 degrees

Therapist: Sitting on the bed facing the patient. Stabilize the patient's leg by placing your right leg on their foot. Grasp the proximal tibia with both hands and place your thumbs on the anterior tibio-femoral joint line.

Action: Apply an anterior translation force to the tibia. Note the end feel and reproduction of symptoms. This test can be repeated with the tibia in internal or external rotation to bias the medial and lateral compartments of the knee.

Stability Test
Tibio-Femoral Joint
Lachman's Test (Anterior Cruciate Ligament)

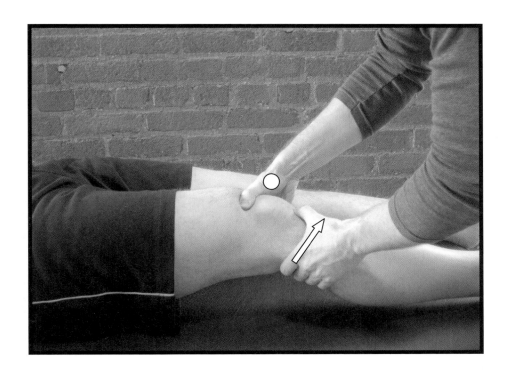

Technique described for the right tibio-femoral joint

Patient: Supine with knee flexed to 30 degrees

Therapist: Standing at the side of the bed. Stabilize the distal femur with your right hand. A rolled towel can also be used to support the femur if your hand is too small. Grasp the proximal tibia with your left hand.

Action: Apply an anterior translation force to the tibia. A positive test may indicate a tear in the anterior cruciate ligament. Note the end feel and reproduction of symptoms.

Stability Test
Tibio-Femoral Joint
Posterior Drawer

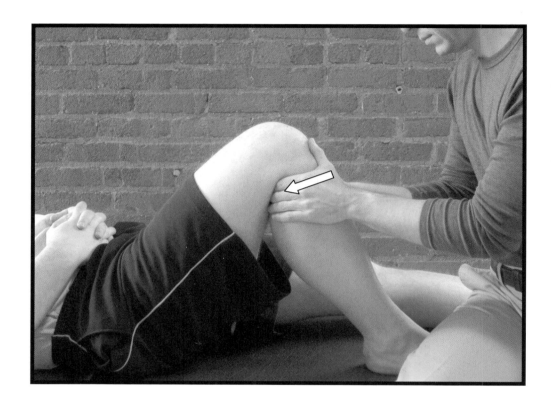

Technique described for the right tibio-femoral joint

Patient: Supine with knee flexed to 90 degrees

Therapist: Sitting on the bed facing the patient. Stabilize the patient's leg by placing your right leg on their foot. Grasp the proximal tibia with both hands and place your thumbs on the anterior tibio-femoral joint line.

Action: Apply a posterior translation force to the tibia. Note the end feel and reproduction of symptoms. This test can be repeated with the tibia in internal or external rotation to bias the medial and lateral compartments of the knee.

Stability Test
Tibio-Femoral Joint
Posterior Sag Test

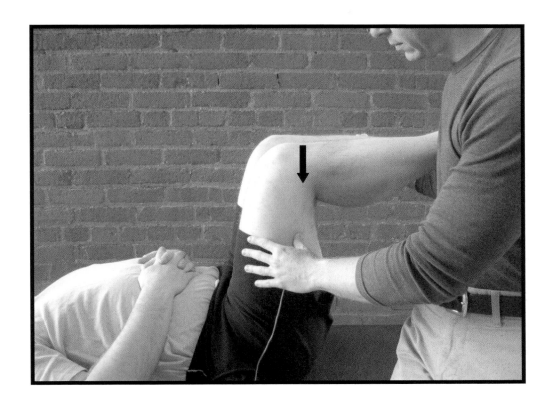

Technique described for the right tibio-femoral joint

Patient: Supine with hips and knees flexed to 90 degrees

Therapist: Standing at the side of the bed. Support the patient's lower legs with your right arm. Make sure the patient's legs are relaxed.

Action: Allow gravity to pull the tibia posteriorly on the femur. Any posterior translation of the right tibia relative to the left indicates a positive test.

Stability Test
Tibio-Femoral Joint
Varus Stress – 0 and 30 degrees

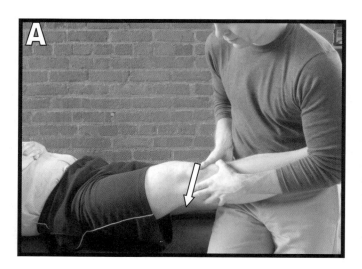
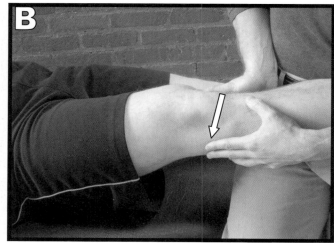

Technique described for the right tibio-femoral joint

Patient: Supine with knee extended

Therapist: Standing at the side of the bed with the patient's right leg cradled between your thorax and left arm. Palpate the lateral collateral ligament with your left index and middle fingers. Place your right hand the medial aspect of the proximal tibia at the tibio-femoral joint line.

Action: Place the knee in extension and apply a varus stress through the tibio-femoral joint with your right hand (A). Repeat with the knee in 30 degrees of flexion (B). Note the end feel and reproduction of symptoms.

Stability Test
Tibio-Femoral Joint
Valgus Stress – 0 and 30 degrees

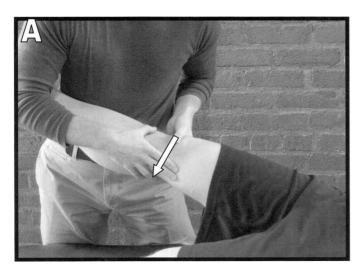 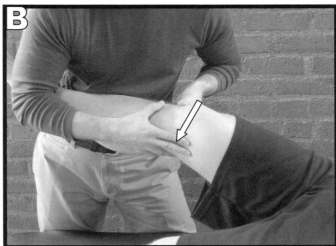

Technique described for the right tibio-femoral joint

Patient: Supine with knee extended

Therapist: Standing at the side of the bed with the patient's right leg cradled between your thorax and right arm. Palpate the medial collateral ligament with your right index and middle fingers. Place your left hand on the lateral aspect of the proximal tibia at the tibio-femoral joint line.

Action: Place the knee in extension and apply a valgus stress through the tibio-femoral joint with your left hand (A). Repeat with the knee in 30 degrees of flexion (B). Note the end feel and reproduction of symptoms.

Stability Test
Tibio-Femoral Joint
Valgus Stress – 90 degrees

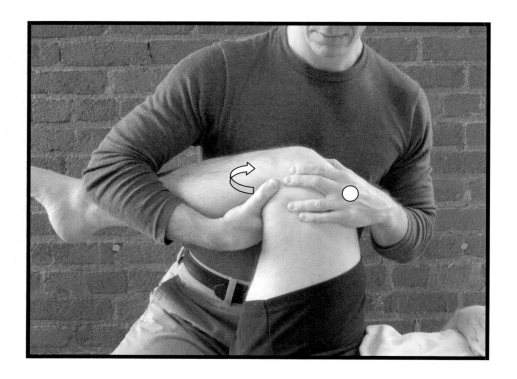

Technique described for the right tibio-femoral joint

Patient: Supine with knee and hip flexed to 90 degrees

Therapist: Standing at the side of the bed with the patient's right leg cradled between your thorax and right arm. Stabilize the distal femur with your left hand while palpating the medial collateral ligament with your index and middle fingers. Place your right hand around the posterior aspect of the proximal tibia at the tibio-femoral joint line.

Action: Apply a valgus stress through the tibio-femoral joint by rotating your body to the right. Note the end feel and reproduction of symptoms.

Meniscal Test
Tibio-Femoral Joint
McMurray's Test

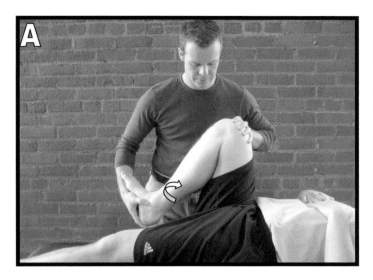 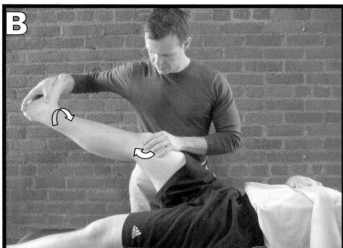

Technique described for the right medial and lateral meniscus

Patient: Supine with hip flexed to 90 degrees and knee fully flexed

Therapist: Standing at the side of the bed. Stabilize the distal femur with your left hand. Grasp the patient's calcaneus with you right hand and use your forearm to hold the talocrural joint in dorsiflexion.

Action: Laterally rotate the tibia in full flexion (A). Passively extend the knee while maintaining the lateral rotation (B). Pain, clicking or locking may indicate a meniscal tear. Repeat with the tibia in medial rotation. Note the end feel and reproduction of symptoms.

Meniscal Test
Tibio-Femoral Joint
Apley's Test

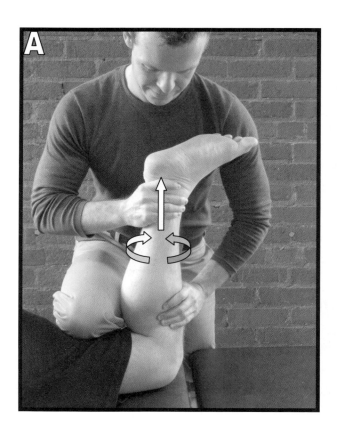 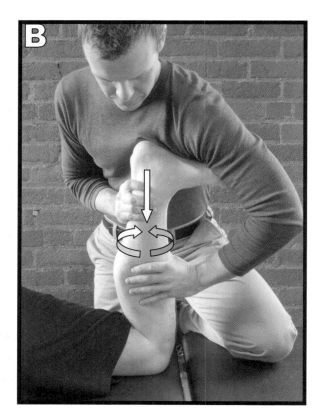

Technique described for the right medial and lateral menisci

Patient: Prone with knee flexed to 90 degrees

Therapist: Standing at the side of the bed. Grasp the proximal tibia with your left hand and the distal tibia with your right hand. Stabilize the femur with your right knee.

Action: Distract the tibio-femoral joint while you medially and laterally rotate the tibia (A). Repeat the test using your body to compress the tibio-femoral joint while you medially and laterally rotate the tibia (B). Note the end feel and reproduction of symptoms.

Meniscal Test
Tibio-Femoral Joint
Joint Line Tenderness

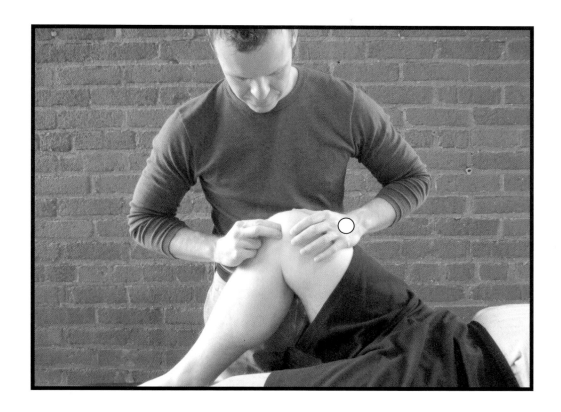

Technique described for the right tibio-femoral joint

Patient: Supine with knee flexed

Therapist: Standing at the side of the bed. Stabilize the distal femur with your left hand. With your right index and middle fingers, palpate the tibio-femoral joint line and the coronary ligaments.

Action: Palpate the anterior-medial and anterior-lateral joint line. Note any reproduction of symptoms.

Stability Test
Patello-Femoral Joint
Traction and Compression

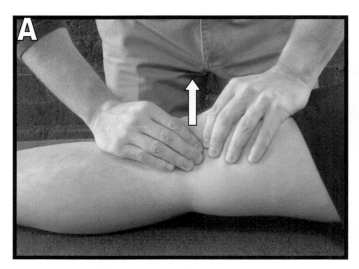 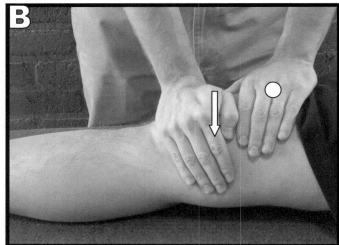

Technique described for the right patella

Patient: Supine with knee extended

Therapist: Standing at the side of the bed. Grasp the distal aspect of the patella with your right thumb and index finger. Grasp the proximal aspect of the patella with your left thumb and index finger.

Action: Apply a traction force to the patella with your right and left hand (A). Note the end feel and reproduction of symptoms. For compression, place the palm of your right hand over the patella and gently compress (B). Note the end feel and reproduction of symptoms.

Stability Test
Patello-Femoral Joint
Superior / Inferior / Medial / Lateral Translation

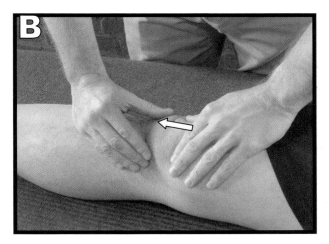

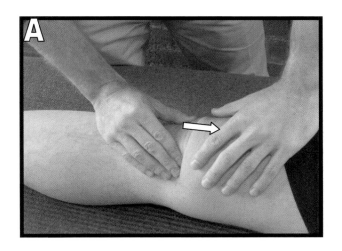

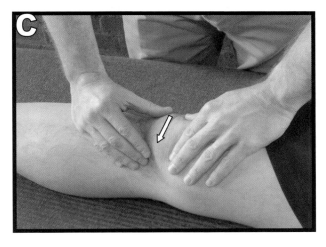

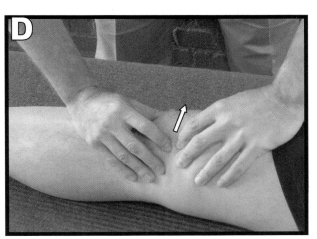

Technique described for the right patella

Patient: Supine with knee extended

Therapist: Standing at the side of the bed. Grasp the distal aspect of the patella with your right thumb and index finger. Grasp the proximal aspect of the patella with your left thumb and index finger.

Action: Apply a superior translation force to the patella with your right hand while controlling the patella with your left hand (A). Note the end feel and reproduction of symptoms. Repeat for inferior translation (B), medial translation (C), and lateral translation (D).

Stability Test
Superior Tibio-Fibular Joint
Compression

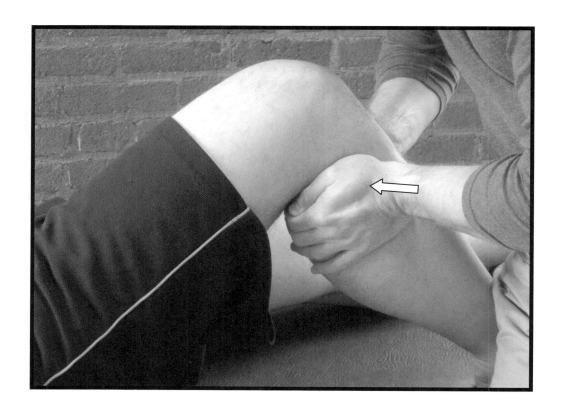

Technique described for the right superior tibio-fibular joint

Patient: Supine with knee flexed to 90 degrees

Therapist: Standing at the side of the bed. Stabilize the proximal tibia with your right hand. Palpate the head of the fibula with the thenar eminence of your left hand.

Action: Apply a compression force to the head of the fibula. Note the end feel and reproduction of symptoms.

Stability Test
Superior Tibio-Fibular Joint
Anterior Translation

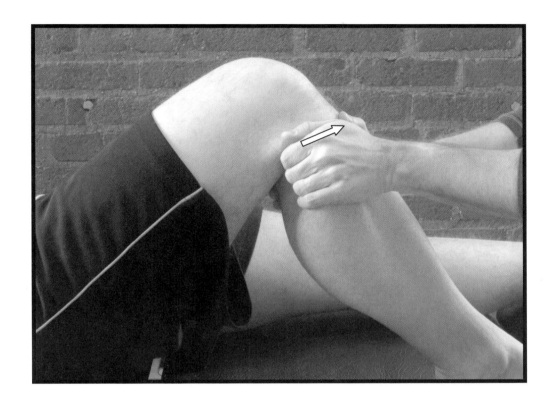

Technique described for the right superior tibio-fibular joint

Patient: Supine with knee flexed to 90 degrees

Therapist: Standing at the side of the bed. Stabilize the proximal tibia with your right hand. Grasp the head of the fibula between the thenar eminence and index and middle fingers of your left hand.

Action: Apply an anterior translation force to the head of the fibula. Note the end feel and reproduction of symptoms.

Stability Test
Superior Tibio-Fibular Joint
Posterior Translation

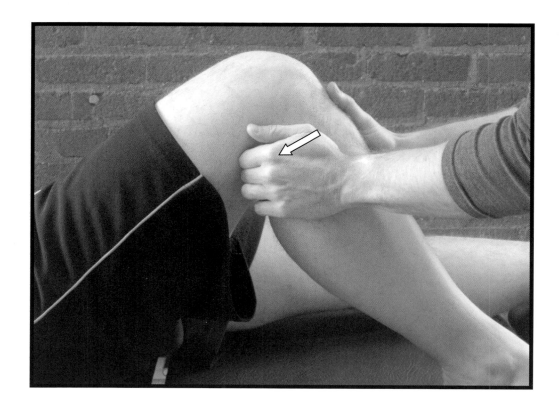

Technique described for the right superior tibio-fibular joint

Patient: Supine with knee flexed to 90 degrees

Therapist: Standing at the side of the bed. Stabilize the proximal tibia with your right hand. Grasp the head of the fibula between the thenar eminence and index and middle fingers of your left hand.

Action: Apply a posterior translation force to the head of the fibula. Note the end feel and reproduction of symptoms.

The Knee
Treatment Techniques

Passive Physiological Mobilization

Passive Accessory Mobilization

Tibiofemoral Joint

Patello-Femoral Joint

Superior Tibio-Fibular Joint

Treatment Technique
Passive Physiological Mobilization
Tibio-Femoral Joint - Flexion

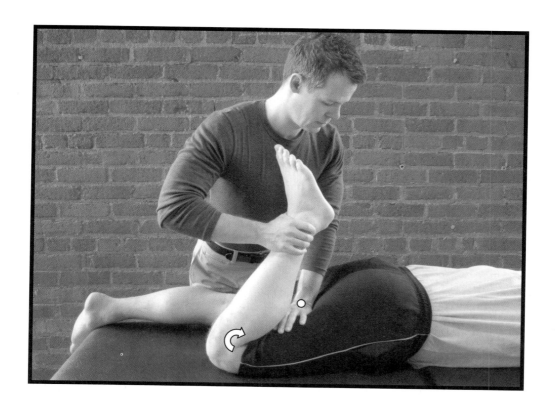

Technique described for the right knee

Indication: Restriction of flexion

Patient: Prone lying with knee flexed

Therapist: Standing at the side of the bed. Stabilize the femur with your left hand while grasping the distal tibia with your right hand.

Action: Mobilize the knee into flexion. At end range, the joint can be biased into the conjunct medial rotation that occurs with flexion. This technique can be graded from 1 to 4.

Treatment Technique
Passive Physiological Mobilization
Tibio-Femoral Joint - Extension

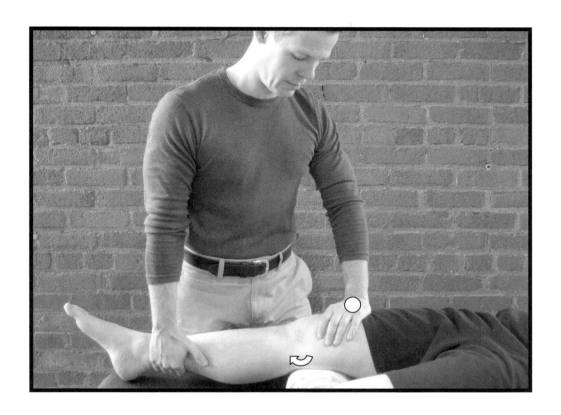

Technique described for the right knee

Indication: Restriction of extension

Patient: Supine lying with a rolled towel under knee

Therapist: Standing at the side of the bed. Stabilize the femur with your left hand while grasping the distal tibia with your right hand.

Action: Mobilize the knee into extension. At end range, the joint can be biased into the conjunct lateral rotation that occurs with extension. This technique can be graded from 1 to 4.

Treatment Technique
Passive Physiological Mobilization
Tibio-Femoral Joint: Combined Flexion-Abduction and Flexion-Adduction

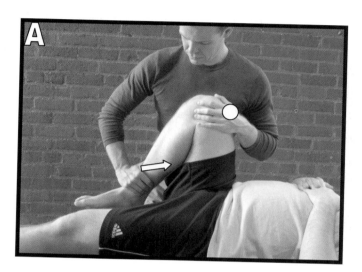 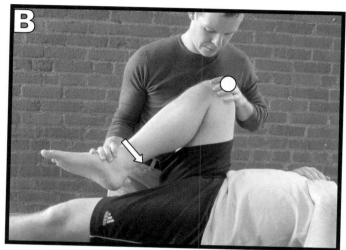

Technique described for right knee

Indication: Restriction of flexion/abduction or flexion/adduction of the knee

Patient: Supine with hip flexed to 90 degrees

Therapist: Standing at the side of the patient. With the left hand, stabilize the distal femur while palpating the tibio-femoral joint line. Grasp the distal tibia with the right hand.

Action: Mobilize the knee joint into flexion/abduction (A) or flexion/adduction (B). Each of the above techniques can be further biased into medial and lateral rotation. These techniques can be graded from 1 to 4.

Treatment Technique

Passive Physiological Mobilization

Tibio-Femoral Joint: Combined Extension-Abduction and Extension-Adduction

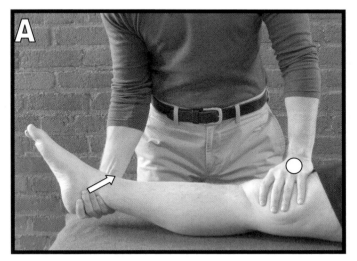 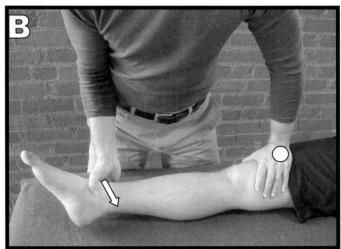

Technique described for right knee

Indication: Restriction of extension/abduction or extension/adduction

Patient: Supine

Therapist: Standing at the side of the patient. With the left hand, stabilize the distal femur while palpating the tibio-femoral joint line. Grasp the distal tibia with the right hand.

Action: Mobilize the knee joint into extension/abduction (A) or extension/adduction (B). Each of the above techniques can be further biased into medial and lateral rotation. These techniques can be graded from 1 to 4.

Treatment Technique
Tibio-Femoral Joint
Anterior Glide

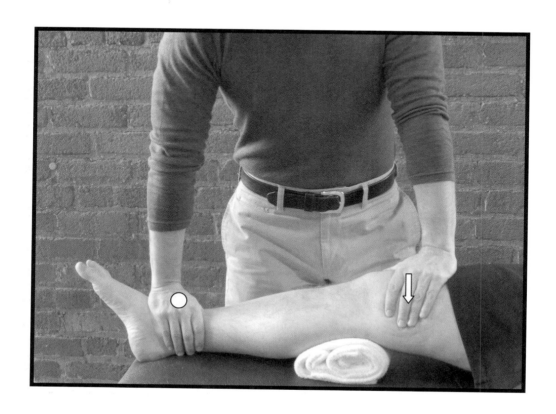

Technique described for the right knee

Indication: Articular restriction of extension

Patient: Supine with a rolled towel under knee

Therapist: Standing at the side of the bed. Stabilize the distal tibia with your right hand. Palpate the anterior aspect of the distal femur with your left hand.

Action: Place the knee in the restriction of extension. Apply a posterior glide to the distal femur. This will produce a relative anterior glide of the tibia. This technique can be graded from 1 to 4.

Treatment Technique
Tibio-Femoral Joint
Posterior Glide

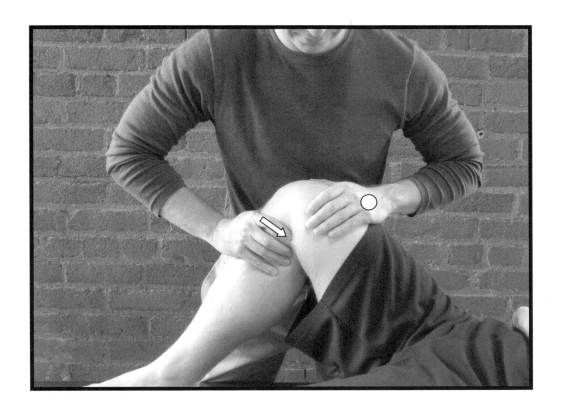

Technique described for the right knee

Indication: Articular restriction of flexion

Patient: Supine lying with knee flexed

Therapist: Standing at the side of the bed. Stabilize the distal femur with your left hand. Palpate the anterior aspect of the proximal tibia with your right hand.

Action: Place the knee in the restriction of flexion. Apply a posterior glide to the tibia. This technique can be graded from 1 to 4.

Treatment Technique
Tibio-Femoral Joint
Medial Glide

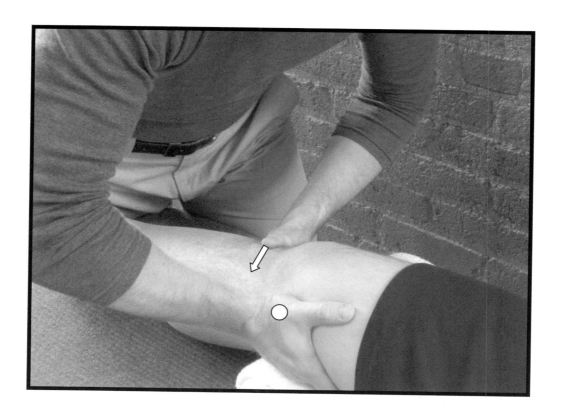

Technique described for the right knee

Indication: Articular restriction of adduction

Patient: Supine with a rolled towel under knee

Therapist: Standing at the side of the bed. Stabilize the medial aspect of the distal femur with your right hand. Palpate the lateral aspect of the proximal tibia with your left hand.

Action: Apply a medial glide to the tibia. This technique can be graded from 1 to 4.

Treatment Technique
Tibio-Femoral Joint
Lateral Glide

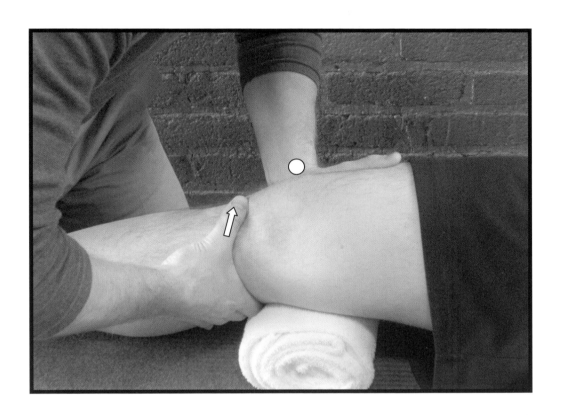

Technique described for the right knee

Indication: Articular restriction of abduction

Patient: Supine with towel roll under knee

Therapist: Standing at the side of the bed. Stabilize the lateral aspect of the distal femur with your left hand. Palpate the medial aspect of the proximal tibia with your right hand.

Action: Apply a lateral glide to the tibia. This technique can be graded from 1 to 4.

Treatment Technique
Patello-Femoral Joint
Superior Glide

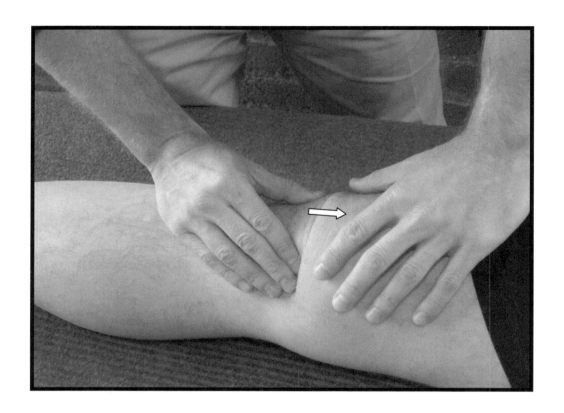

Technique described for the right patella

Indication: A superior glide restriction of the patella

Patient: Supine with knee extended

Therapist: Standing at the side of the bed. Grasp the distal aspect of the patella with your right thumb and index finger. Grasp the proximal aspect of the patella with your left thumb and index finger.

Action: Apply a superior glide to the patella with your right hand while controlling the patella with your left hand. This technique can be graded from 1 to 4.

Treatment Technique
Patello-Femoral Joint
Inferior Glide

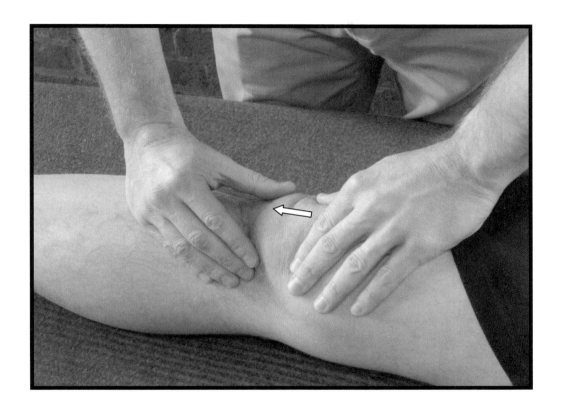

Technique described for the right patella

Indication: An inferior glide restriction of the patella

Patient: Supine with knee extended

Therapist: Standing at the side of the bed. Grasp the distal aspect of the patella with your right thumb and index finger. Grasp the proximal aspect of the patella with your left thumb and index finger.

Action: Apply an inferior glide to the patella with your left hand while controlling the patella with your right hand. This technique can be graded from 1 to 4.

Treatment Technique
Patello-Femoral Joint
Medial Glide

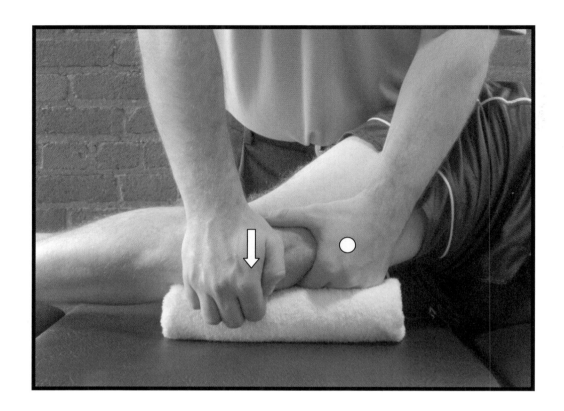

Technique described for the right patella

Indication: A medial glide restriction of the patella

Patient: Left side lying with knee slightly flexed and a rolled towel under knee

Therapist: Standing at the side of the bed. Stabilize the medial aspect of the distal femur with your left hand. Palpate the lateral aspect of the patella with the heel of your right hand.

Action: Apply a medial glide to the patella with your right hand. This technique can be graded from 1 to 4.

Treatment Technique
Patello-Femoral Joint
Lateral Glide

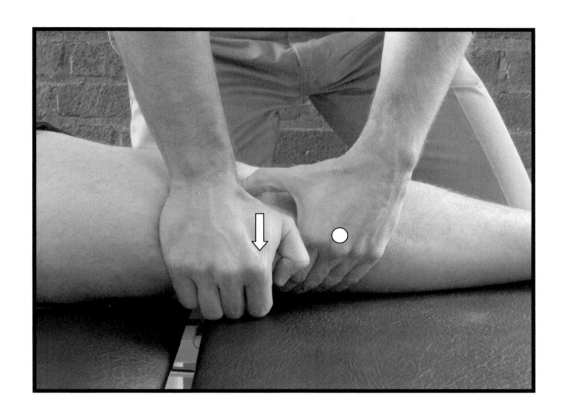

Technique described for the right patella

Indication: A lateral glide restriction of the patella.

Patient: Right side lying with knee slightly flexed

Therapist: Standing at the side of the bed. Stabilize the lateral aspect of the proximal tibia with your left hand. Palpate the medial aspect of the patella with the heel of your right hand.

Action: Apply a lateral glide to the patella with your right hand. This technique can be graded from 1 to 4.

Treatment Technique
Superior Tibio-Fibular Joint
Anterior Glide

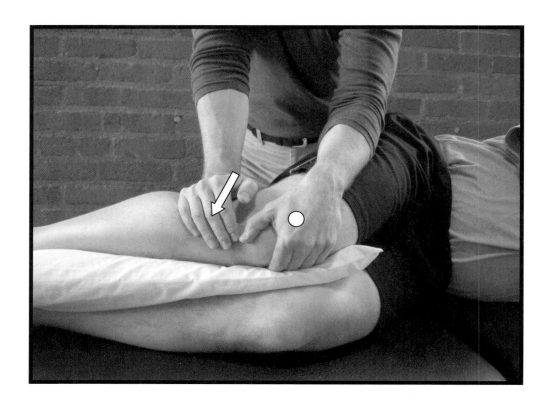

Technique described for the right superior tibio-fibular joint

Indication: An anterior glide restriction of the fibula

Patient: Left side lying with knees flexed and pillow between them

Therapist: Standing at the side of the bed. Stabilize the distal femur with your left hand. Palpate the head of the fibula with the heel of your right hand.

Action: Apply an anterior glide to the fibula with your right hand. This technique can be graded from 1 to 4.

Treatment Technique
Superior Tibio-Fibular Joint
Posterior Glide

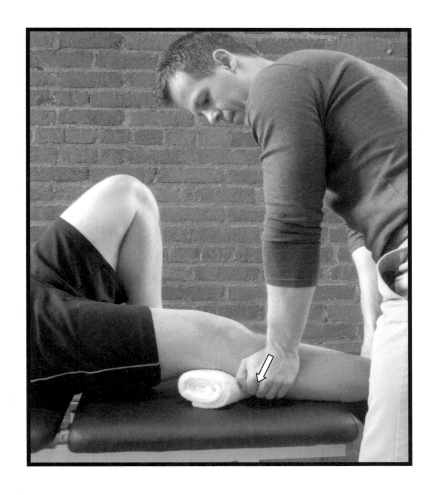

Technique described for the right superior tibio-fibular joint

Indication: A posterior glide restriction of the fibula

Patient: Supine with a rolled towel under knee

Therapist: Standing at the end of the bed. Stabilize the distal tibia and fibula with your right hand. Palpate the head of the fibula with the heel of your left hand.

Action: Apply a posterior glide to the head of the fibula. This technique can be graded from 1 to 4.

The Talocrural Joint

The Talocrural Joint
Active and Passive Movement Testing

Weight Bearing Range of Motion
Squat - Dorsiflexion

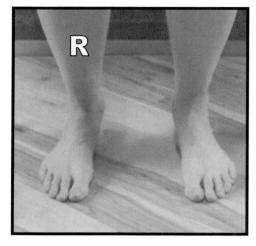

Front

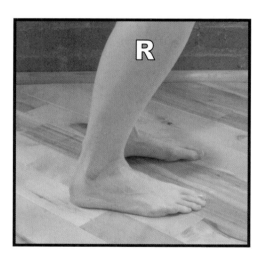

Back

Side

Technique described for the right ankle

Patient: Standing with feet flat on floor pointing straight ahead

Therapist: Crouching in front of patient

Action: Instruct the patient to perform a half squat. Observe the range of motion and note any reproduction of symptoms. Repeat while observing from the side and back.

Active Range of Motion
Heel Raise - Plantarflexion

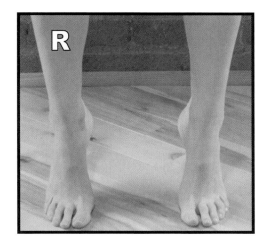

Front

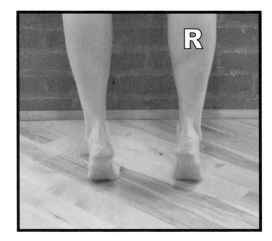

Back

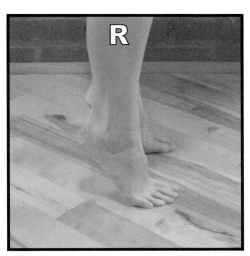

Side

Technique described for the right ankle

Patient: Standing with feet pointing straight ahead

Therapist: Crouching in front of patient

Action: Instruct the patient to rise up on their toes. Observe the range of motion and note any reproduction of symptoms. Repeat while observing from the side and back.

Passive Range of Motion
Dorsiflexion

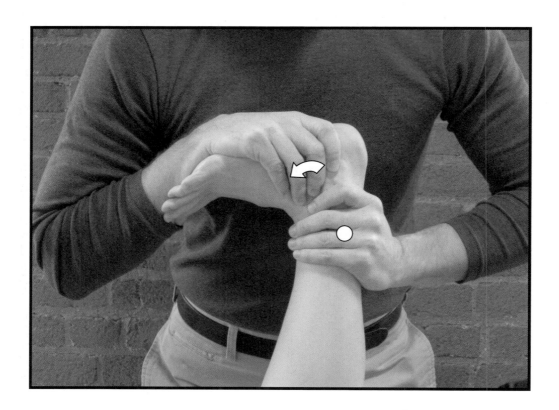

Technique described for the right ankle

Patient: Prone lying with knee flexed

Therapist: Standing at the side of the bed. Stabilize the distal tibia and fibula with your left hand. Grasp the hindfoot and midfoot with your right hand.

Action: Passively dorsiflex the talocrural joint. Note the range of motion, end feel and reproduction of symptoms.

Passive Range of Motion
Plantarflexion

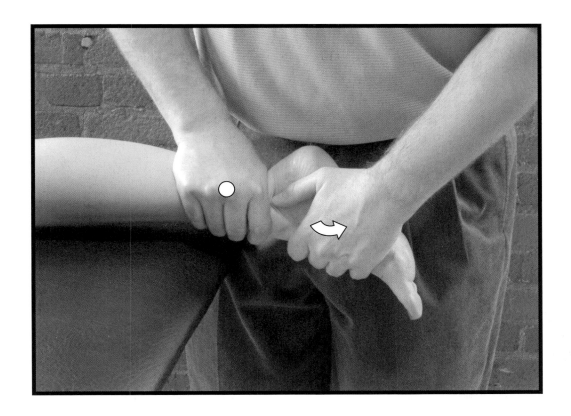

Technique described for the right ankle

Patient: Prone lying with foot off the edge of bed

Therapist: Standing at the side of the bed. Stabilize the distal tibia and fibula with your right hand. Grasp the anterior aspect of the talus and midfoot with your left hand.

Action: Passively plantarflex the talocrural joint. Note the range of motion, end feel and reproduction of symptoms.

Passive Range of Motion
Talar Swing

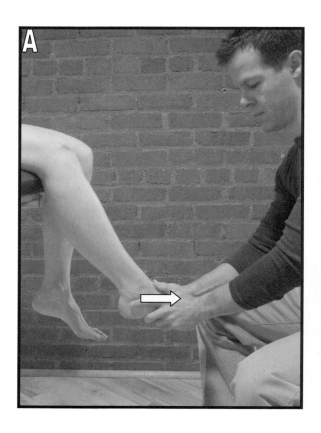
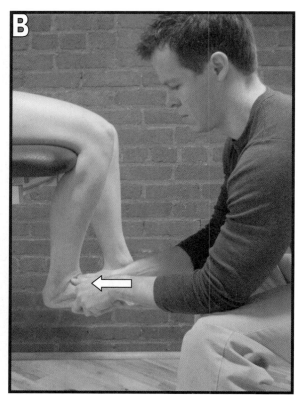

Technique described for the right ankle

Patient: Sitting at end of bed knees at 90 degrees

Therapist: Sitting in front of the patient. Grasp the patient's foot with both hands while palpating the anterior joint line of the talus with your thumbs.

Action: Passively plantarflex (A) and dorsiflex (B) the talocrural joint. Note the range of motion, end feel and reproduction of symptoms.

Passive Accessory Motion
Posterior Glide

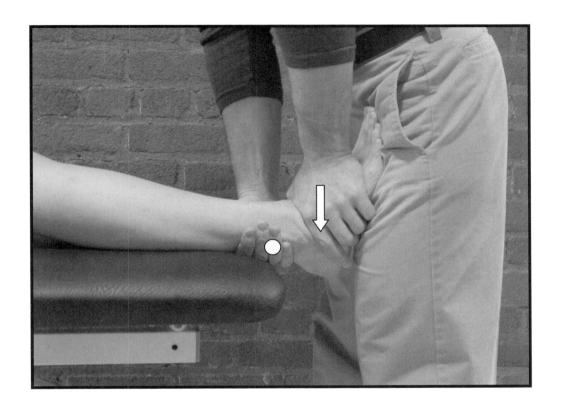

Technique described for the right ankle

Patient: Supine lying foot over end of bed with the talocrural joint in neutral

Therapist: Standing at the end of the bed with the patient's foot resting on your left thigh. Stabilize the tibia and fibula with your right hand. Grasp the anterior aspect of the talus with your left hand.

Action: Apply a posterior force to the talus. Note the range of motion, end feel and reproduction of symptoms.

Passive Accessory Motion
Anterior Glide

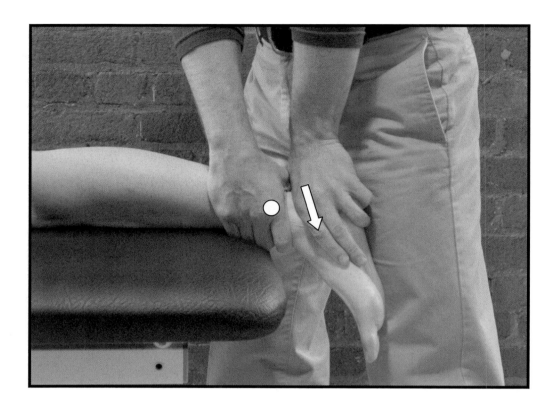

Technique described for the right ankle

Patient: Prone lying, foot over end of bed with the talocrural joint in neutral

Therapist: Standing at the end of the bed. Stabilize the tibia and fibula with your right hand. Grasp the posterior aspect of the talus and calcaneus with your left hand.

Action: Apply an anterior force to the talus. Note the range of motion, end feel and reproduction of symptoms.

Passive Accessory Motion
Inferior Tibio-fibular Joint
Anterior Glide

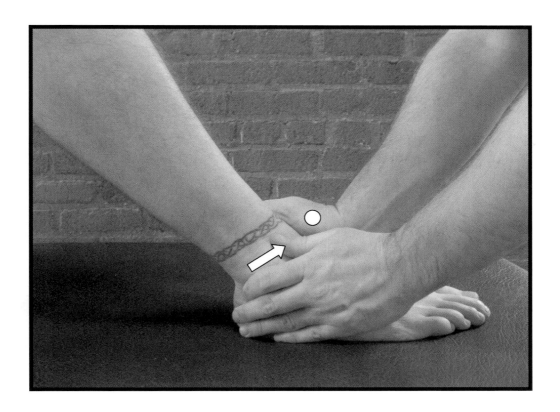

Technique described for the right ankle

Patient: Crook lying with right foot flat on bed

Therapist: Standing at the end of the bed. Stabilize the medial malleolus with your right hand. Grasp the lateral malleolus with your left hand.

Action: Apply an anterior force to the lateral malleolus. Note the range of motion, end feel and reproduction of symptoms.

Passive Accessory Motion
Inferior Tibio-Fibular Joint
Posterior Glide

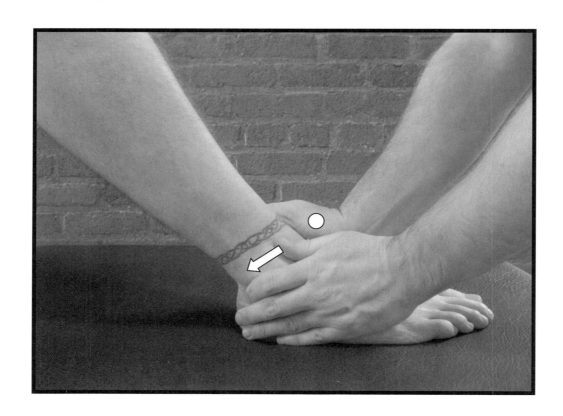

Technique described for the right ankle

Patient: Crook lying with right foot flat on bed

Therapist: Standing at the end of the bed. Stabilize the medial malleolus with your right hand. Grasp the lateral malleolus with your left hand.

Action: Apply a posterior force to the lateral malleolus. Note the range of motion, end feel and reproduction of symptoms.

The Talocrural Joint
Stability Tests

Talocrural Joint

Inferior Tibio-Fibular Joint

Stability Test
Traction

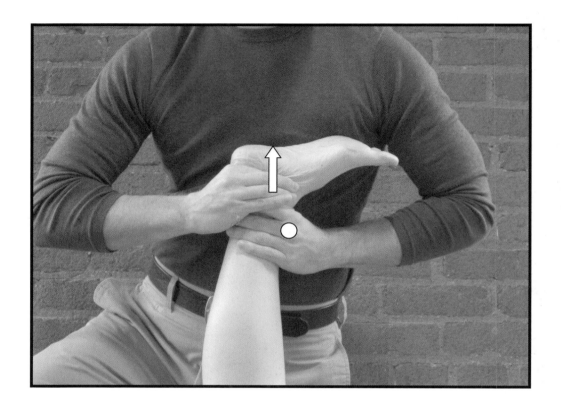

Technique described for the right ankle

Patient: Prone lying with knee flexed to 90 degrees

Therapist: Standing at the side of the bed. Stabilize the distal tibia and fibula with your left hand. Grasp the talus with the right hand.

Action: Apply a traction force to the talus. Note the end feel and reproduction of symptoms.

Stability Test
Compression

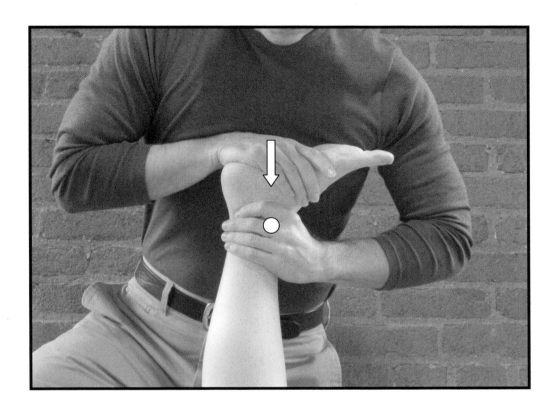

Technique described for the right ankle

Patient: Prone lying with knee flexed to 90 degrees

Therapist: Standing at the side of the bed. Stabilize the distal tibia and fibula with your left hand. Place the palm of your right hand on the plantar surface of the calcaneus.

Action: Apply a compression force through the calcaneus. Note the end feel and reproduction of symptoms.

Stability Test
Anterior Drawer

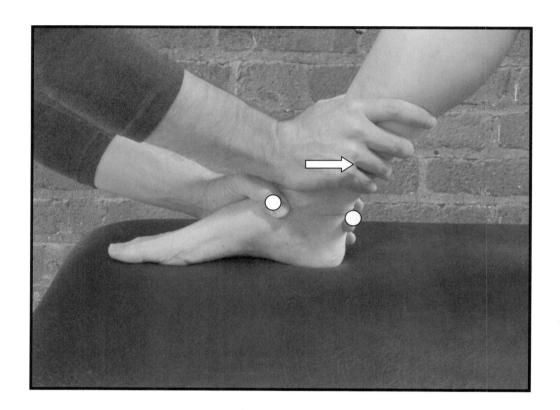

Technique described for the right ankle

Patient: Crook lying with foot flat on bed

Therapist: Standing at the end of the bed. Stabilize the talus with your left hand.
Grasp the anterior aspect of the distal tibia and fibula with your right hand.

Action: Apply a posterior translation force to the distal tibia and fibula, parallel to the
talocrural joint surface, while stabilizing the talus. This will create a relative anterior
translation of the talus in the ankle mortise. Note the end feel and reproduction of
symptoms.

Stability Test
Posterior Drawer

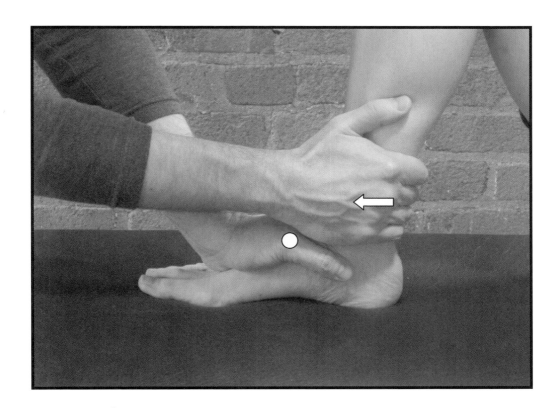

Technique described for the right ankle

Patient: Crook lying with foot flat on bed

Therapist: Standing at the end of the bed. Stabilize the talus with your left hand. Grasp the posterior aspect of the distal tibia and fibula with your right hand.

Action: Apply an anterior translation force to the distal tibia and fibula, parallel to the talocrural joint surface, while stabilizing the talus. This will create a relative posterior translation of the talus in the ankle mortise. Note the end feel and reproduction of symptoms.

Ligament Stress Test
Anterior Talofibular Ligament

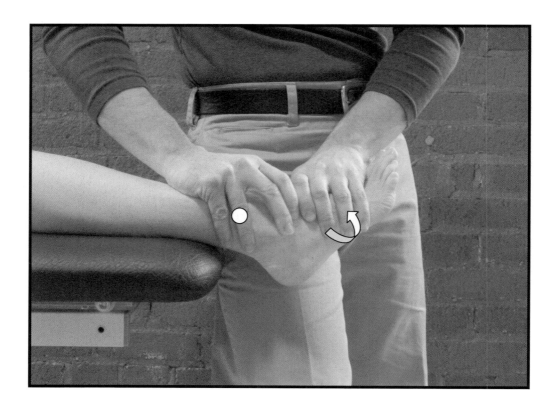

Technique described for the right ankle

Patient: Supine lying with right foot over end of bed

Therapist: Standing at the end of the bed. Stabilize the distal tibia and fibula with your right hand while palpating the anterior talofibular ligament with your right index finger. Grasp the talus with your left hand.

Action: Plantarflex and invert the talocrural joint and apply a varus force to the talus. Note the end feel and reproduction of symptoms.

Ligament Stress Test
Calcaneofibular Ligament

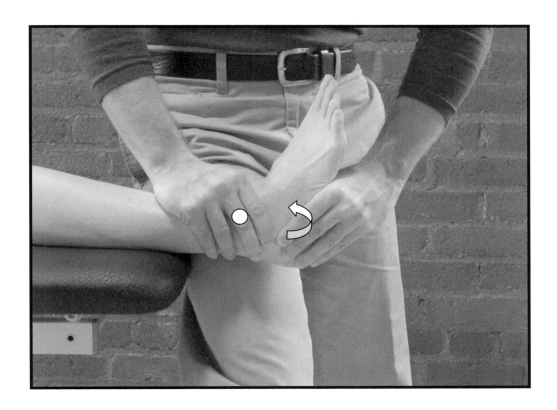

Technique described for the right ankle

Patient: Supine lying with right foot over end of bed

Therapist: Standing at the end of the bed. Stabilize the distal tibia and fibula with your right hand while palpating the calcaneofibular ligament with your right index finger. Grasp the calcaneus with your left hand.

Action: Place the talocrural joint in inversion and neutral dorsiflexion and apply a varus force to the talus. Note the end feel and reproduction of symptoms.

Ligament Stress Test
Posterior Talofibular Ligament

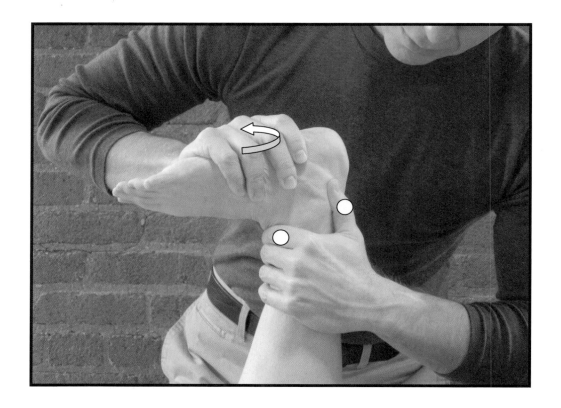

Technique described for the right ankle

Patient: Prone lying with knee flexed to 90 degrees

Therapist: Standing at side of the bed. Stabilize the distal tibia and fibula with your left hand. Grasp the plantar aspect of the foot with your right hand.

Action: Dorsiflex the talocrural joint to end range. Invert the talus and apply an external rotation force. Note the end feel and reproduction of symptoms.

Ligament Stress Test
Deltoid Ligament – Anterior Band

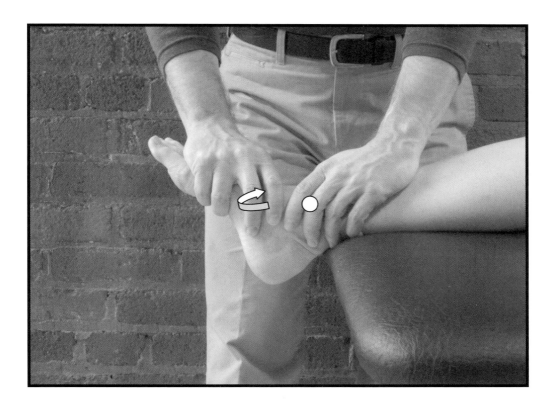

Technique described for the right ankle

Patient: Supine lying with right foot over end of bed

Therapist: Standing at the end of the bed. Stabilize the distal tibia and fibula with your left hand while palpating the anterior band of the deltoid ligament with your left index finger. Grasp the anterior aspect of the talus with your right hand.

Action: Position the talocrural joint in plantarflexion and eversion and apply a valgus force to the talus. Note the end feel and reproduction of symptoms.

Ligament Stress Test
Deltoid Ligament – Middle Band

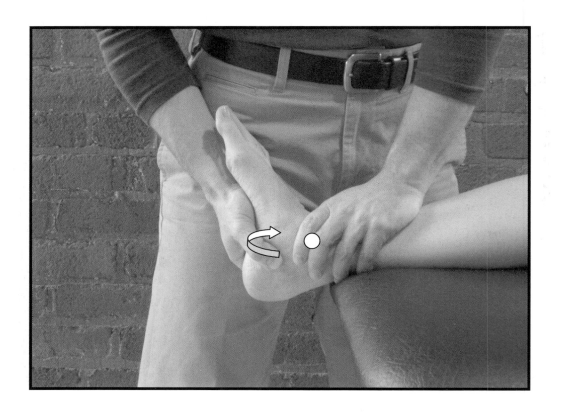

Technique described for the right ankle

Patient: Supine lying with right foot over end of bed

Therapist: Standing at the end of the bed. Stabilize the distal tibia and fibula with your left hand while palpating the middle band of the deltoid ligament with your left index finger. Grasp the calcaneus with your right hand.

Action: Position the talocrural joint in eversion and neutral dorsiflexion and apply a valgus force to the talus. Note the end feel and reproduction of symptoms.

Ligament Stress Test
Deltoid Ligament – Posterior Band

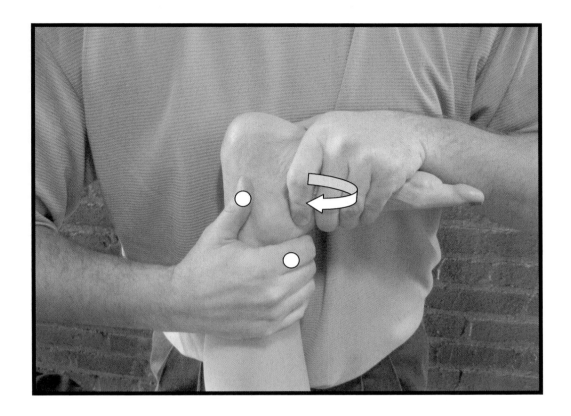

Technique described for the right ankle

Patient: Prone lying with knee flexed to 90 degrees

Therapist: Standing at the side of the bed. Stabilize the tibia with your right hand. Grasp the plantar aspect of the foot with left hand.

Action: Dorsiflex the talocrural joint to end range. Evert the talus and apply an internal rotation force. Note the end feel and reproduction of symptoms.

Stability Test
Inferior Tibio-Fibular Joint
Weight Bearing Dorsiflexion (Mortise Splay)

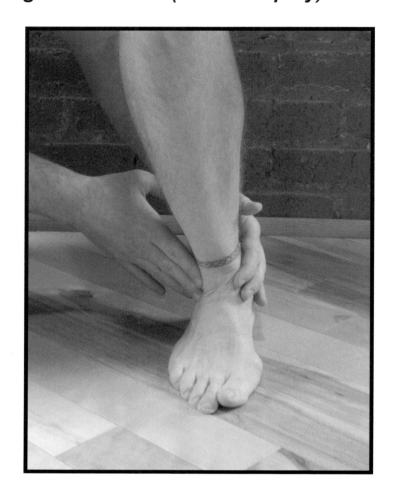

Technique described for the right ankle

Patient: Standing

Therapist: Crouched beside the patient. Palpate the anterior aspect of the medial malleolus with your left hand and the anterior aspect of the lateral malleolus with your right hand.

Action: Instruct the patient to perform a partial squat. Palpate for splaying of the inferior tibio-fibular joint. Note the range of motion and reproduction of symptoms.

The Talocrural Joint
Treatment Techniques

Passive Physiological Mobilization

Passive Accessory Mobilization

Inferior Tibio-Fibular Joint

Treatment Technique
Passive Physiological Mobilization
Dorsiflexion

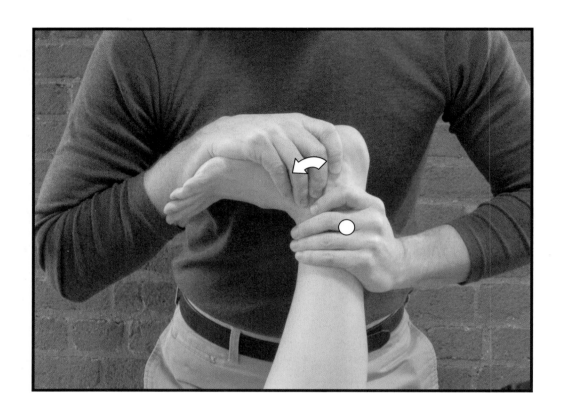

Technique described for the right ankle

Indication: Restriction of dorsiflexion

Patient: Prone with knee flexed to 90 degrees

Therapist: Standing at the side of the bed. Stabilize the distal tibia and fibula with your left hand. Grasp the foot and talus with your right hand.

Action: Mobilize the talocrural joint into dorsiflexion. This technique can be graded from 1 to 4.

Treatment Technique
Passive Physiological Mobilization
Plantarflexion

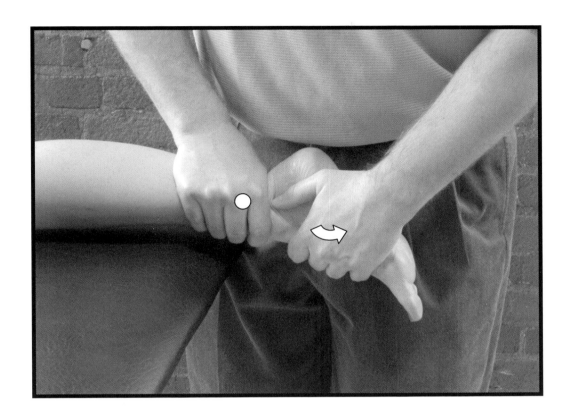

Technique described for the right ankle

Indication: Restriction of plantarflexion

Patient: Prone lying with foot off the edge of bed

Therapist: Standing at the side of the bed. Stabilize the distal tibia and fibula with your right hand. Grasp the anterior aspect of the talus and midfoot with your left hand.

Action: Mobilize the talocrural joint into plantarflexion. This technique can be graded from 1 to 4.

Treatment Technique
Traction

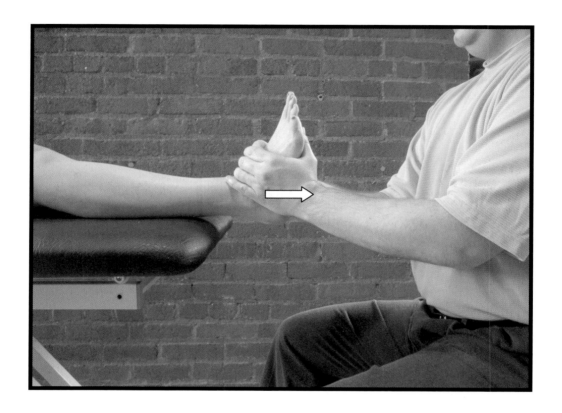

Technique described for the right ankle

Indication: Articular restriction of the talocrural joint

Patient: Supine lying with foot over end of bed

Therapist: Sitting on a stool at the end of the bed. With both hands, grasp the patient's foot at the talocrural joint line. Keep your elbows close together.

Action: Apply a traction force to the talus by shifting your weight backward. This technique can be graded 1 to 4.

Treatment Technique
Traction With Belt (Alternate Technique)

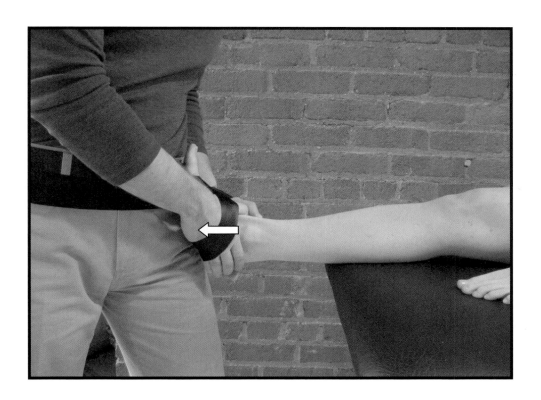

Technique described for the right ankle

Indication: Articular restriction of the talocrural joint

Patient: Supine lying with foot over end of bed

Therapist: Standing at the end of the bed. Place a mobilizing belt around your waist and the patient's ankle. Place your hands through the mobilization belt and grasp the talus.

Action: Apply a traction force to the talus through the belt by shifting your weight onto your back leg. This technique can be graded 1 to 4.

Treatment Technique
Posterior Glide

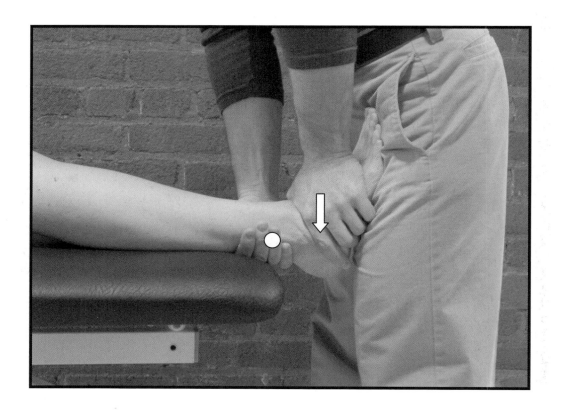

Technique described for the right ankle

Indication: Articular restriction of dorsiflexion

Patient: Supine lying with foot over end of bed

Therapist: Stand facing the patient with their foot resting on your left thigh. Stabilize the distal tibia and fibula with your right hand. Grasp the anterior aspect of the talus with your left hand.

Action: Place the talocrural joint in the restriction of dorsiflexion. Apply a posterior glide to the talus. This technique can be graded from 1 to 4.

Treatment Technique
Posterior Glide
(Alternate Technique)

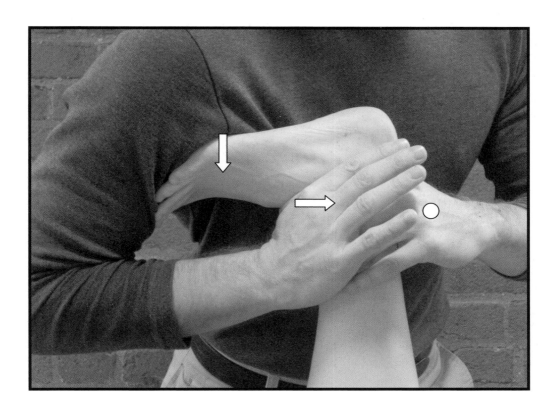

Technique described for the right ankle

Indication: Articular restriction of dorsiflexion

Patient: Prone lying with knee flexed

Therapist: Standing at the side of the bed. Stabilize the distal tibia and fibula with your left hand. Grasp the anterior aspect of the talus with your right hand while dorsiflexing the foot with your right shoulder.

Action: Apply a posterior glide to the talus while maintaining dorsiflexion with your right shoulder. This technique can be graded from1 to 4.

Treatment Technique
Anterior Glide

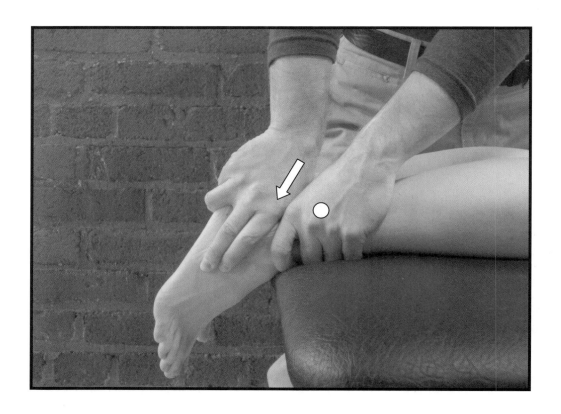

Technique described for the right ankle

Indication: Articular restriction of plantarflexion

Patient: Prone lying with foot over end of bed

Therapist: Standing at the end of the bed. Stabilize the distal tibia and fibula with your left hand. Grasp the posterior aspect of the talus with your right hand.

Action: Place the talocrural joint in the restriction of plantarflexion. Apply an anterior glide to the talus. This technique can be graded from1 to 4.

Treatment Technique
Inferior Tibio-fibular Joint
Anterior Glide

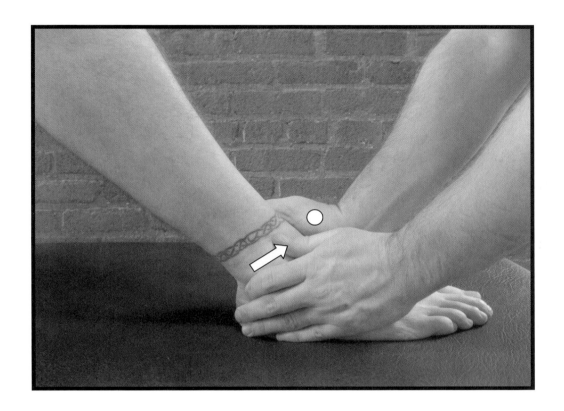

Technique described for the right ankle

Indication: Articular restriction of the inferior tibio-fibular joint

Patient: Crook lying with right foot flat on bed

Therapist: Standing at the end of the bed. Stabilize the medial malleolus with your right hand. Grasp the lateral malleolus with your left hand.

Action: Apply an anterior glide to the lateral malleolus. This technique can be graded from 1 to 4.

Treatment Technique
Inferior Tibio-Fibular Joint
Posterior Glide

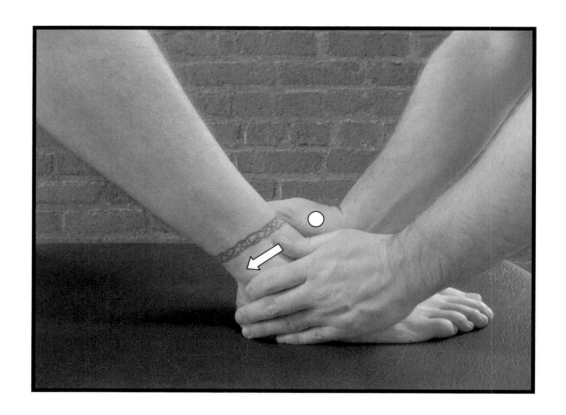

Technique described for the right ankle

Indication: Articular restriction of the inferior tibio-fibular joint

Patient: Crook lying with right foot flat on bed

Therapist: Standing at the end of the bed. Stabilize the medial malleolus with your right hand. Grasp the lateral malleolus with your left hand.

Action: Apply a posterior glide to the lateral malleolus. This technique can be graded from 1 to 4.

The Subtalar Joint

The Subtalar Joint
Active and Passive Movement Testing

Weight Bearing Range of Motion

Passive Range of Motion

Passive Accessory Motions

Weight Bearing Range of Motion
Supination (Heel Raise and Body Twist)

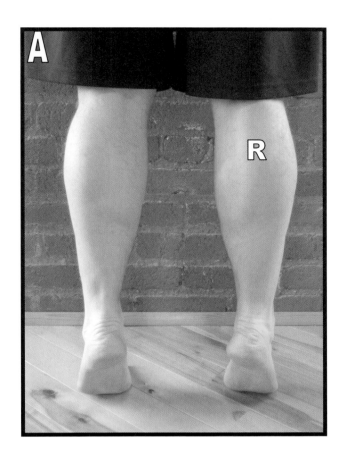 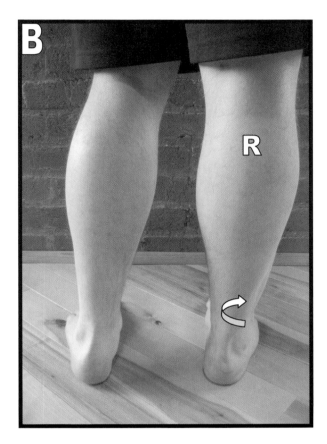

Technique described for the right subtalar joint

Patient: Standing with feet pointing straight ahead

Therapist: Crouching behind the patient

Action: Instruct the patient to rise up on their toes (A). Instruct the patient to body twist to the right (B). Observe the range of motion in the subtalar joint and note any reproduction of symptoms.

Weight Bearing Range of Motion
Pronation (Squat and Body Twist)

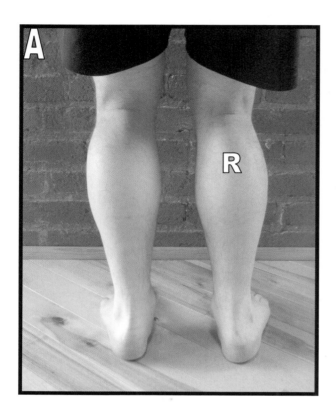 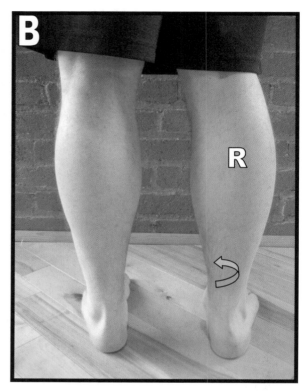

Technique described for the right subtalar joint

Patient: Standing with feet pointing straight ahead

Therapist: Crouching behind the patient

Action: Instruct the patient to perform a half squat (A). Instruct the patient to body twist to the left (B). Observe the range of motion in the subtalar joint and note any reproduction of symptoms.

Passive Range of Motion
Supination

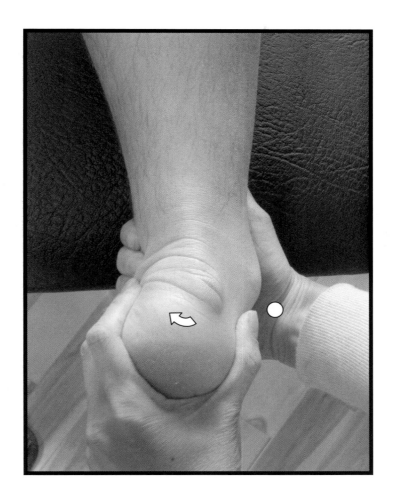

Technique described for the right subtalar joint

Patient: Prone lying with foot over end of bed

Therapist: Standing at the end of the bed. Stabilize the anterior aspect of the talus with your right hand. Grasp the calcaneus with your left hand.

Action: Passively supinate the subtalar joint. Note the range of motion, end feel and reproduction of symptoms.

Passive Range of Motion
Pronation

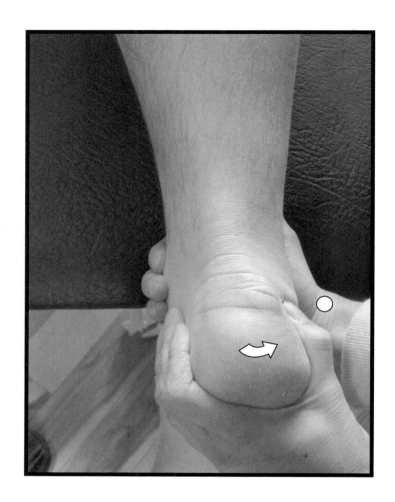

Technique described for the right subtalar joint

Patient: Prone lying with foot over end of bed

Therapist: Standing at the end of the bed. Stabilize the anterior aspect of the talus with your right hand. Grasp the calcaneus with your left hand.

Action: Passively pronate the subtalar joint. Note the range of motion, end feel and reproduction of symptoms.

Passive Accessory Motion
Anterior Joint Medial Glide

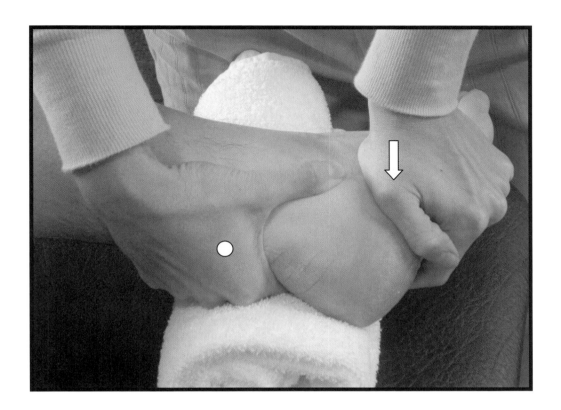

Technique described for the right subtalar joint

Patient: Left side lying with a rolled towel placed under medial malleolus

Therapist: Standing at the end of the bed. Stabilize the posterior aspect of the talus with your right hand. Place the heel of your left hand on the anterior-lateral aspect of the calcaneus.

Action: Apply a medial force to the calcaneus. Note the range of motion, end feel and reproduction of symptoms.

Passive Accessory Motion
Anterior Joint Lateral Glide

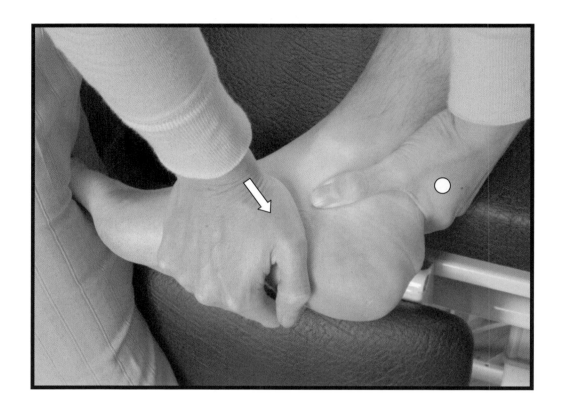

Technique described for the right subtalar joint

Patient: Right side lying with foot off edge of bed

Therapist: Standing at the end of the bed. Stabilize the posterior aspect of the talus with your left hand. Place the heel of your right hand on the anterior-medial aspect of the calcaneus.

Action: Apply a lateral force to the calcaneus. Note the range of motion, end feel and reproduction of symptoms.

Passive Accessory Motion
Posterior Joint Medial Glide

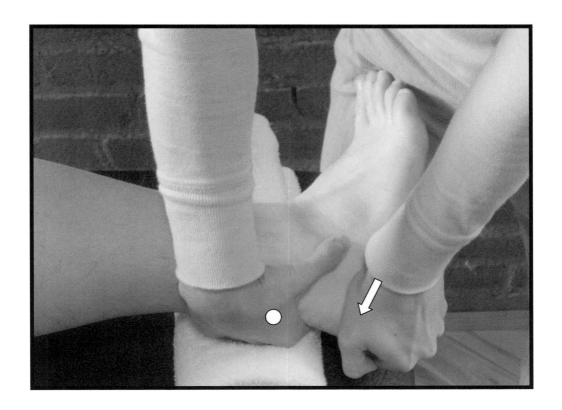

Technique described for the right subtalar joint

Patient: Left side lying with a rolled towel placed under medial malleolus

Therapist: Standing at the end of the bed. Stabilize the posterior aspect of the talus with your right hand. Place the heel of your left hand on the posterior-lateral aspect of the calcaneus.

Action: Apply a medial force to the calcaneus. Note the range of motion, end feel and reproduction of symptoms.

Passive Accessory Motion
Posterior Joint Lateral Glide

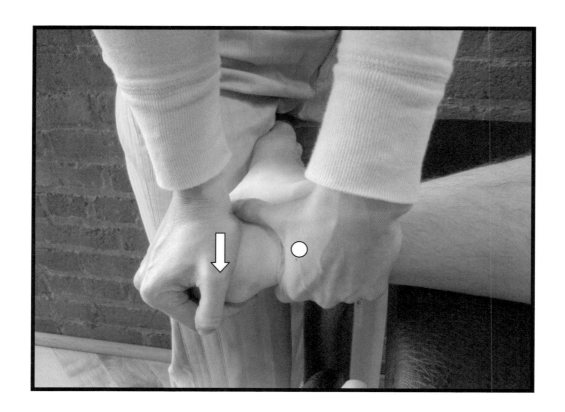

Technique described for the right subtalar joint

Patient: Right side lying with foot off edge of bed

Therapist: Standing at the end of the bed. Stabilize the posterior aspect of the talus with your left hand. Place the heel of your right hand on the posterior-medial aspect of the calcaneus.

Action: Apply a lateral force to the calcaneus. Note the range of motion, end feel and reproduction of symptoms.

The Subtalar Joint
Passive Stability Tests

Passive Stability Test
Compression

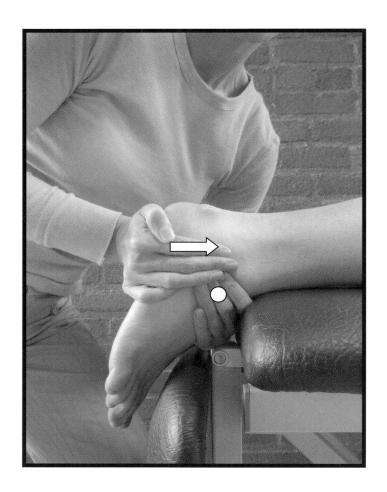

Technique described for the right subtalar joint

Patient: Prone lying with foot off end of bed

Therapist: Standing at the end of the bed. Stabilize the anterior aspect of the talus with your left hand. Place the palm of your right hand over the plantar aspect of the calcaneus.

Action: Apply a compressive force through the calcaneus. Note the end feel and reproduction of symptoms.

Passive Stability Test
Traction

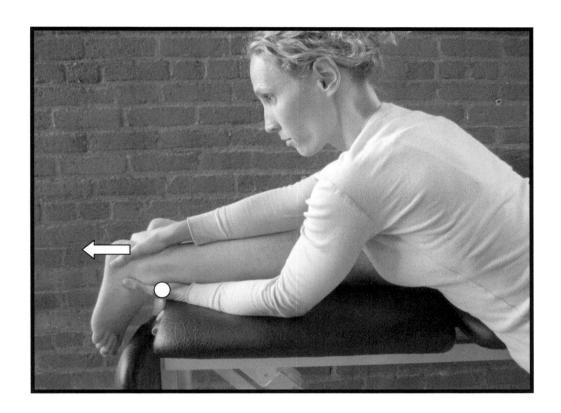

Technique described for the right subtalar joint

Patient: Prone lying with foot off end of bed

Therapist: Standing at the side of the bed. Stabilize the anterior aspect of the talus with your left hand. Grasp the posterior aspect of the calcaneus with your right hand.

Action: Apply a traction force to the calcaneus. Note the end feel and reproduction of symptoms.

Ligament Stress Test
Medial Talocalcaneal and Interosseus Ligaments

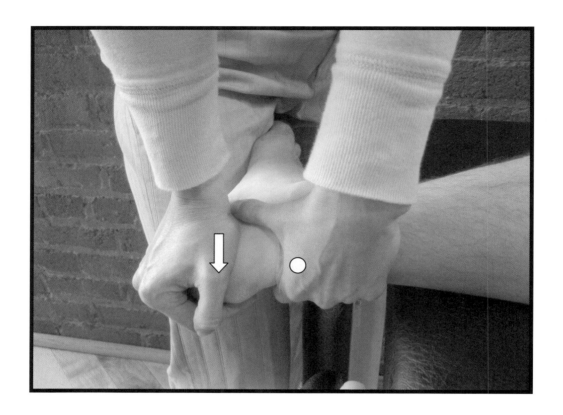

Technique described for the right subtalar joint

Patient: Right side lying with foot off edge of bed

Therapist: Standing at the end of the bed. Stabilize the posterior aspect of the talus with your left hand. Place the heel of your right hand on the medial aspect of the calcaneus.

Action: Passively pronate the subtalar joint and apply a lateral translation force to the calcaneus. This will stress the medial talocalcaneal and interosseus ligaments. Note the end feel and reproduction of symptoms.

Ligament Stress Test
Lateral Talocalcaneal and Cervical Ligaments

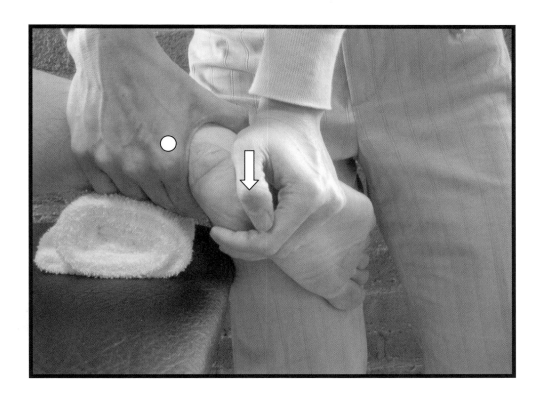

Technique described for the right subtalar joint

Patient: Left side lying with a rolled towel placed under medial malleolus

Therapist: Standing at the side of the bed. Stabilize the posterior aspect of the talus with your right hand. Place the heel of your left hand on the lateral aspect of the calcaneus.

Action: Passively supinate the subtalar joint and apply a medial translation force to the calcaneus. This will stress the lateral talocalcaneal and cervical ligament. Note the end feel and reproduction of symptoms.

The Subtalar Joint
Treatment Techniques

Passive Physiological Mobilization

Treatment Technique

Passive Physiological Mobilization
Supination

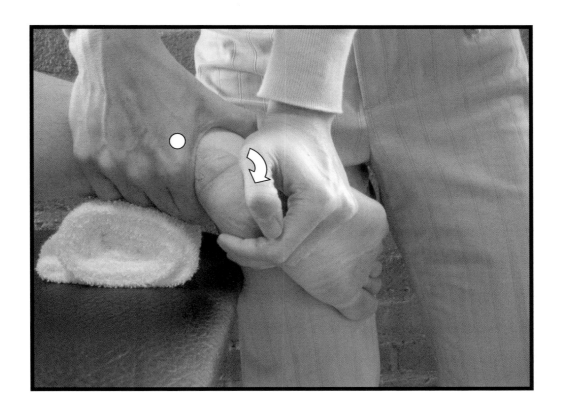

Technique described for the right subtalar joint

Indication: Restriction of supination

Patient: Left side lying with a rolled towel placed under medial malleolus

Therapist: Standing at the end of the bed. Stabilize the posterior aspect of the talus with your right hand. Place the heel of your left hand on the lateral aspect of the calcaneus.

Action: Mobilize the subtalar joint into supination. This technique can be graded form 1 to 4.

Treatment Technique

Passive Physiological Mobilization
Pronation

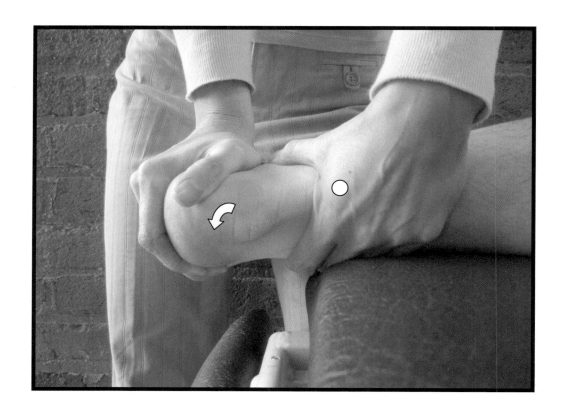

Technique described for the right subtalar joint

Indication: Restriction of pronation

Patient: Right side lying with foot off edge of bed

Therapist: Standing at the end of the bed. Stabilize the posterior aspect of the talus with your left hand. Place the heel of your right hand on the medial aspect of the calcaneus.

Action: Mobilize the subtalar joint into pronation. This technique can be graded from 1 to 4.

Treatment Technique
Traction

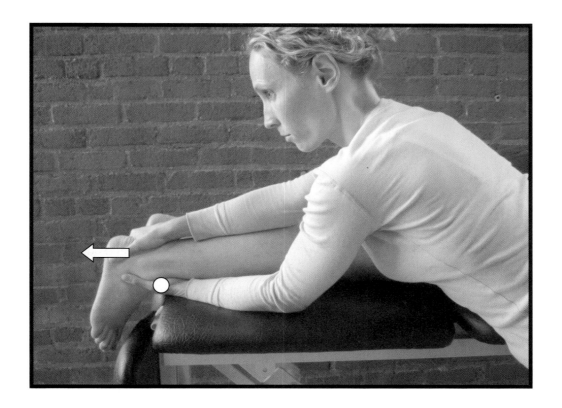

Technique described for the right subtalar joint

Indication: Articular restriction of the subtalar joint

Patient: Prone lying with foot off end of bed

Therapist: Standing at the side of the bed. Stabilize the anterior aspect of the talus with your left hand. Grasp the posterior aspect of the calcaneus with your right hand.

Action: Apply a traction force to the calcaneus. This technique can be graded from 1 to 4.

Treatment Technique
Anterior Joint Lateral Glide

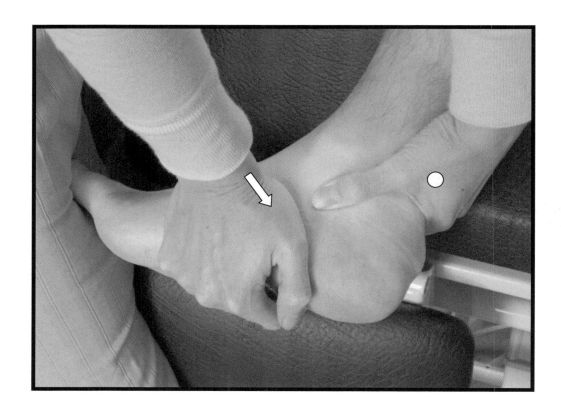

Technique described for the right subtalar joint

Indication: Articular restriction of pronation at the anterior subtalar joint

Patient: Right side lying with foot off edge of bed

Therapist: Standing at the end of the bed. Stabilize the posterior aspect of the talus with your left hand. Place the heel of your right hand on the anterior-medial aspect of the calcaneus.

Action: Position the subtalar joint into the restriction of pronation and apply a lateral glide to the calcaneus. This technique can be graded from 1 to 4.

Treatment Technique
Anterior Joint Medial Glide

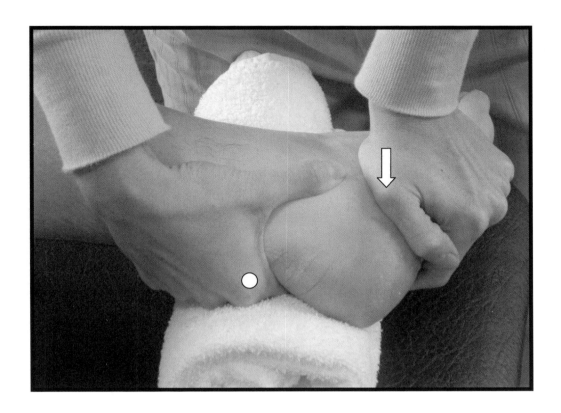

Technique described for the right subtalar joint

Indication: Articular restriction of supination at the anterior subtalar joint

Patient: Left side lying with a rolled towel placed under medial malleolus

Therapist: Standing at the side of the bed. Stabilize the posterior aspect of the talus with your right hand. Place the heel of your left hand on the anterior-lateral aspect of the calcaneus.

Action: Position the subtalar joint into the restriction of supination and apply a medial glide to the calcaneus. This technique can be graded from 1 to 4.

Treatment Technique
Posterior Joint Lateral Glide

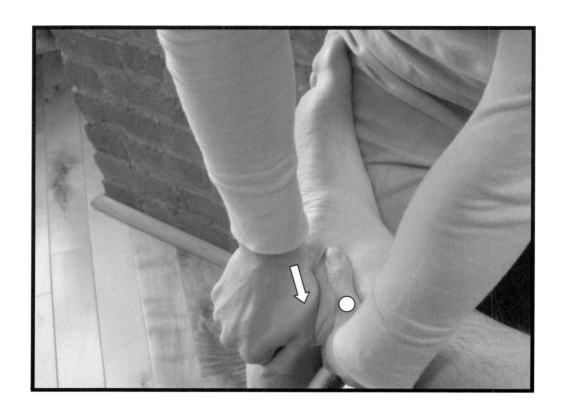

Technique described for the right subtalar joint

Indication: Articular restriction of supination at the posterior subtalar joint

Patient: Right side lying with foot off edge of bed

Therapist: Standing at the end of the bed. Stabilize the posterior aspect of the talus with your left hand. Place the heel of your right hand on the posterior-medial aspect of the calcaneus.

Action: Position the subtalar joint into the restriction of supination and apply a lateral glide to the calcaneus. This technique can be graded from 1 to 4.

Treatment Technique
Posterior Joint Medial Glide

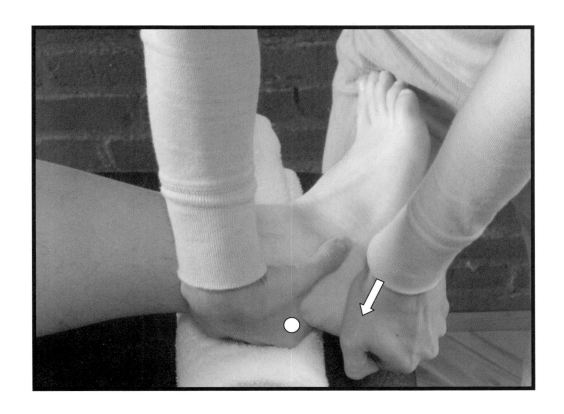

Technique described for the right subtalar joint

Indication: Articular restriction of pronation at the posterior subtalar joint

Patient: Left side lying with a rolled towel placed under the medial malleolus

Therapist: Standing at the end of the bed. Stabilize the posterior aspect of the talus with your right hand. Place the heel of your left hand on the posterior-lateral aspect of the calcaneus.

Action: Position the subtalar joint into the restriction of pronation and apply a medial glide to the calcaneus. This technique can be graded from 1 to 4.

The Midfoot

The Midfoot
Active and Passive Movement Testing

Weight Bearing Range of Motion

Passive Range of Motion

Passive Accessory Motion

Weight Bearing Range of Motion
Pronation
(Body Twist and Squat)

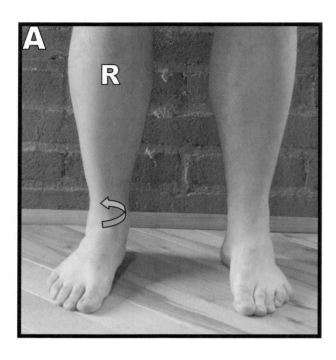
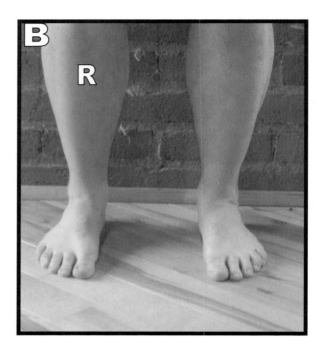

Technique described for the right midfoot

Patient: Standing with feet pointing straight ahead

Therapist: Crouching in front of the patient

Action: Instruct the patient to twist to the left (A). Instruct the patient to partially squat while keeping their heels on the ground (B). Observe the range of motion in the midfoot and note any reproduction of symptoms. These two movements will cause the right midfoot to pronate.

Weight Bearing Range of Motion
Supination
(Body Twist and Up on Toes)

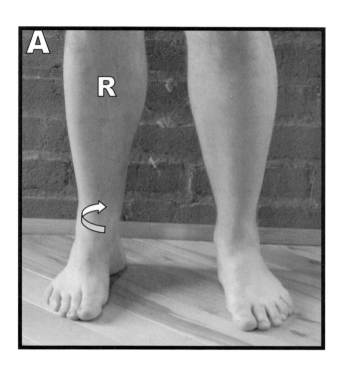
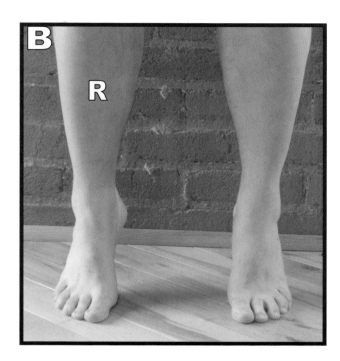

Technique described for the right midfoot

Patient: Standing with feet pointing straight ahead

Therapist: Crouching in front of the patient

Action: Instruct the patient to twist to the right (A). Instruct the patient to raise up on their toes (B). Observe the range of motion in the midfoot and note any reproduction of symptoms. These two movements will cause the right midfoot to supinate.

Passive Range of Motion
Pronation
(Dorsiflexion-Abduction-Eversion)

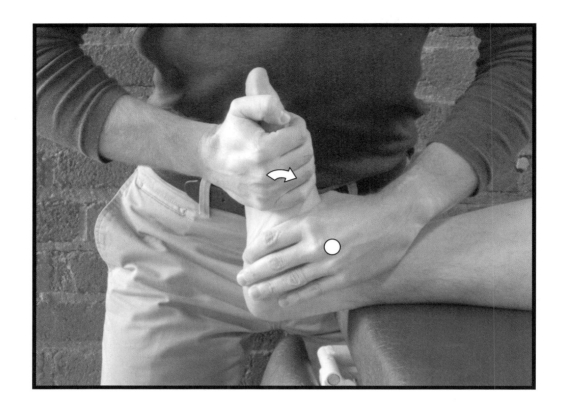

Technique described for the right midfoot

Patient: Supine lying with foot off edge of bed

Therapist: Standing at the end of the bed. Stabilize the talus and calcaneus with your left hand. Grasp the sole of the foot with your right hand.

Action: Passively pronate the patient's midfoot (dorsiflexion-abduction-eversion). Note the range of motion, end feel and reproduction of symptoms.

Passive Range of Motion
Supination
(Plantarflexion-Adduction-Inversion)

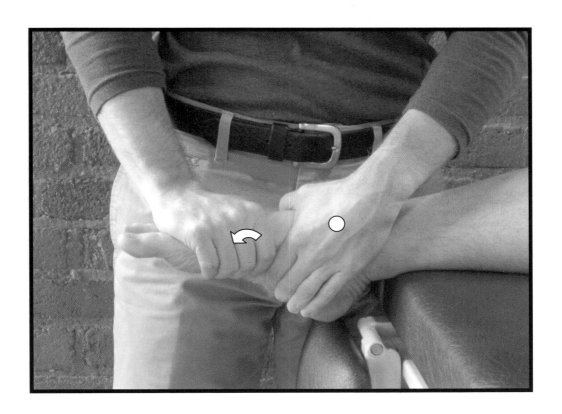

Technique described for the right midfoot

Patient: Supine lying with foot off edge of bed

Therapist: Standing at the end of the bed. Stabilize the talus and calcaneus with your left hand. Grasp the forefoot with the right hand.

Action: Passively supinate the patient's midfoot (plantarflexion-adduction-inversion). Note the range of motion, end feel and reproduction of symptoms.

Passive Range of Motion
Fanning

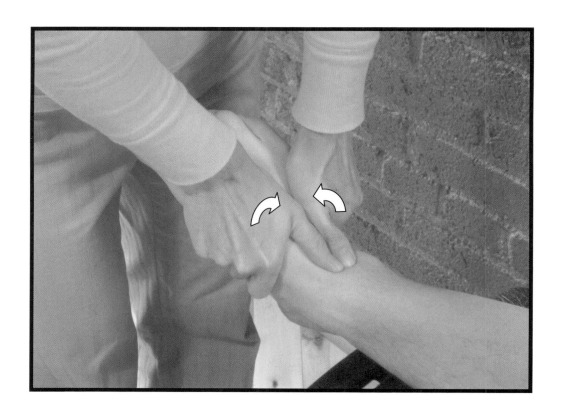

Technique described for the right midfoot

Patient: Supine lying with foot off edge of bed

Therapist: Standing at the end of the bed. Grasp the foot with both hands, placing your thumbs along the midline.

Action: Passively fan the patient's foot by moving the medial and lateral borders of the midfoot in a dorsal direction. Note the range of motion, end feel and reproduction of symptoms.

Passive Range of Motion
Folding

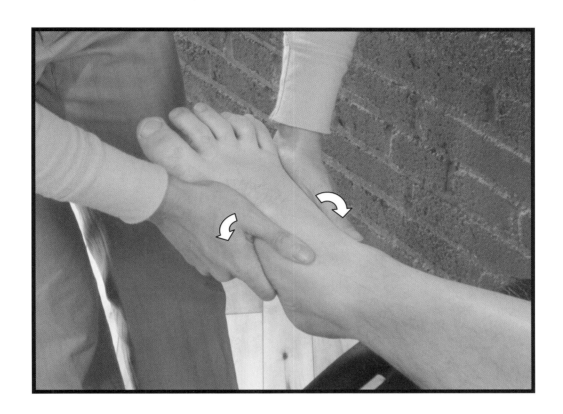

Technique described for the right midfoot

Patient: Supine lying with foot off edge of bed

Therapist: Standing at the end of the bed. Grasp the foot with both hands, placing your thumbs along the midline.

Action: Passively fold the patient's foot by moving the medial and lateral borders of the midfoot in a plantar direction. Note the range of motion, end feel and reproduction of symptoms.

Passive Accessory Motion
Talonavicular Dorsal Glide

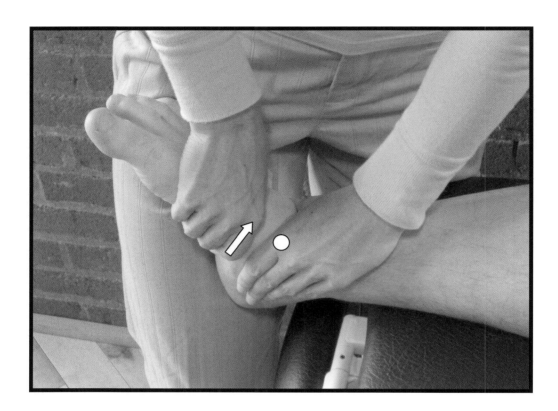

Technique described for the right talonavicular joint

Patient: Supine lying with foot off edge of bed

Therapist: Standing at the end of the bed. Stabilize the head of the talus with your left hand. Grasp the navicular with your right hand.

Action: Apply a dorsal force to the navicular allowing the conjunct external rotation to occur. Note the range of motion, end feel and reproduction of symptoms.

Passive Accessory Motion
Talonavicular Plantar Glide

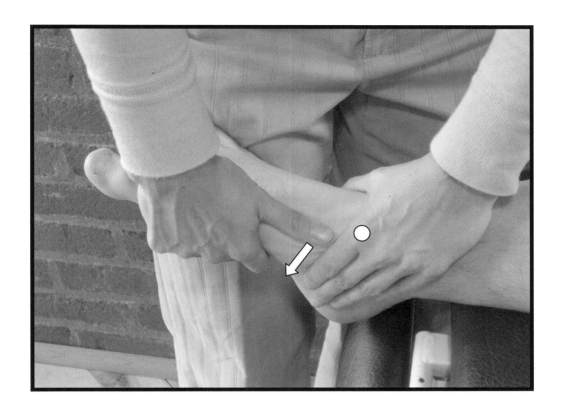

Technique described for the right talonavicular joint

Patient: Supine lying with foot off edge of bed

Therapist: Standing at the end of the bed. Stabilize the head of the talus with your left hand. Grasp the navicular with your right index finger and thumb.

Action: Apply a plantar force to the navicular allowing the conjunct internal rotation to occur. Note the range of motion, end feel and reproduction of symptoms

Passive Accessory Motion
Calcaneocuboid Dorsal Glide

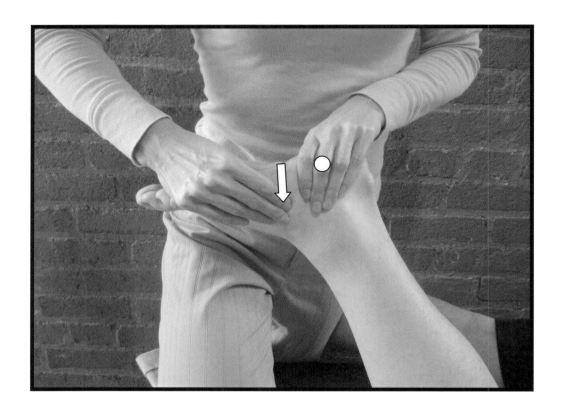

Technique described for the right calcaneocuboid joint

Patient: Prone lying with the knee flexed

Therapist: Standing at the side of the bed. Stabilize the calcaneus with your left hand. Grasp the cuboid with your right index finger and thumb.

Action: Apply a dorsal force to the cuboid allowing the conjunct internal rotation and abduction to occur. Note the range of motion, end feel and reproduction of symptoms.

Passive Accessory Motion
Calcaneocuboid Plantar Glide

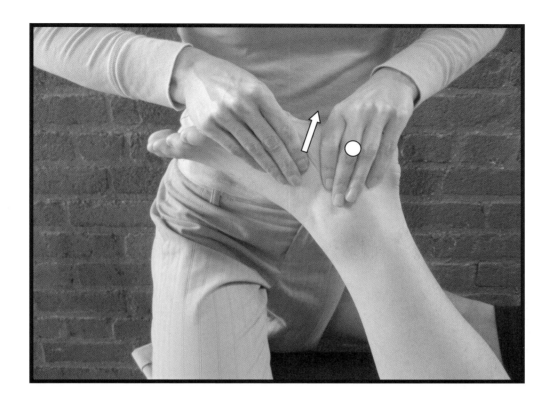

Technique described for the right calcaneocuboid joint

Patient: Prone lying with the knee flexed

Therapist: Standing at the side of the bed. Stabilize the calcaneus with your left hand. Grasp the cuboid with your right index finger and thumb.

Action: Apply a plantar force to the cuboid allowing the conjunct external rotation and adduction to occur. Note the range of motion, end feel and reproduction of symptoms.

Passive Accessory Motion
Cuneonavicular Joint Dorsal Glide

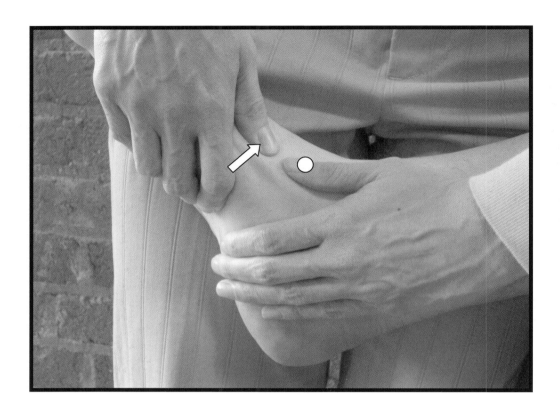

Technique described for the right cuneonavicular joint

Patient: Supine lying with foot off edge of bed

Therapist: Standing at the end of the bed. Stabilize the navicular with your left hand. Grasp the medial cuneiform with your right index finger and thumb.

Action: Apply a dorsal force to the medial cuneiform allowing the conjunct external rotation to occur. Note the range of motion, end feel and reproduction of symptoms.

Passive Accessory Motion
Cuneonavicular Joint Plantar Glide

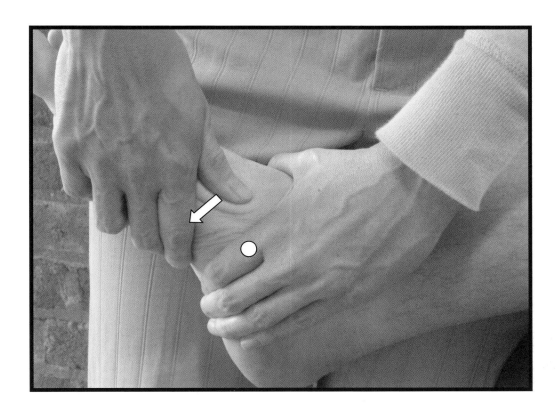

Technique described for the right cuneonavicular joint

Patient: Supine lying with foot off edge of bed

Therapist: Standing at the end of the bed. Stabilize the navicular with your left hand. Grasp the medial cuneiform with your right index finger and thumb.

Action: Apply a plantar force to the medial cuneiform allowing the conjunct internal rotation to occur. Note the range of motion, end feel and reproduction of symptoms.

Passive Accessory Motion
Cuneocuboid Joint Dorsal Glide

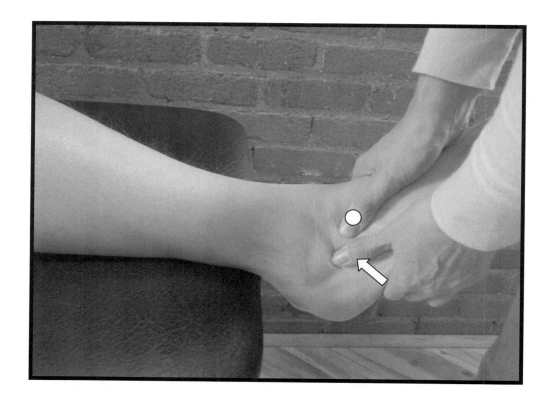

Technique described for the right cuneocuboid joint

Patient: Supine lying with foot off edge of bed

Therapist: Standing at the end of the bed. Stabilize the lateral cuneiform with your right hand. Grasp the cuboid with your left index finger and thumb.

Action: Apply a dorsal force to the cuboid. Note the range of motion, end feel and reproduction of symptoms.

Passive Accessory Motion
Cuneocuboid Joint Plantar Glide

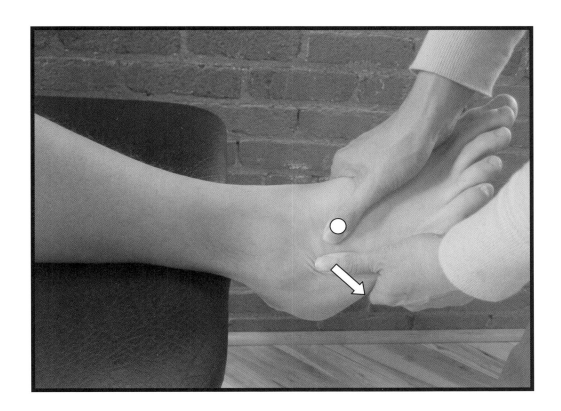

Technique described for the right cuneocuboid joint

Patient: Supine lying with foot off edge of bed

Therapist: Standing at the end of the bed. Stabilize the lateral cuneiform with your right hand. Grasp the cuboid with your left index finger and thumb.

Action: Apply a plantar force to the cuboid. Note the range of motion, end feel and reproduction of symptoms.

Passive Accessory Motion
Intercuneiform Joint Dorsal Glide

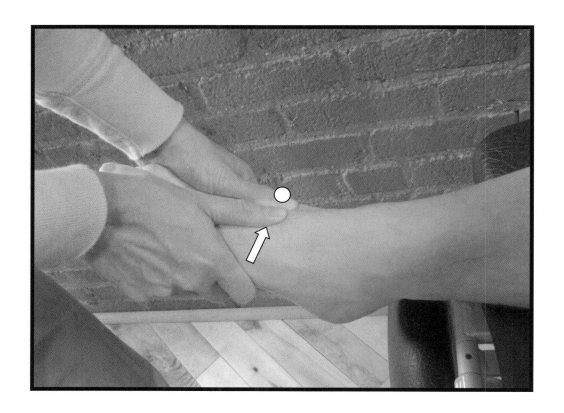

Technique described for the right medial intercuneiform joint

Patient: Supine lying with foot off edge of bed

Therapist: Standing at the end of the bed. Stabilize the middle cuneiform with your left hand. Grasp the medial cuneiform with your right index finger and thumb.

Action: Apply a dorsal force to the medial cuneiform. Note the range of motion, end feel and reproduction of symptoms. Repeat the technique for a dorsal glide of the lateral cuneiform on the middle cuneiform.

Passive Accessory Motion
Intercuneiform Joint Plantar Glide

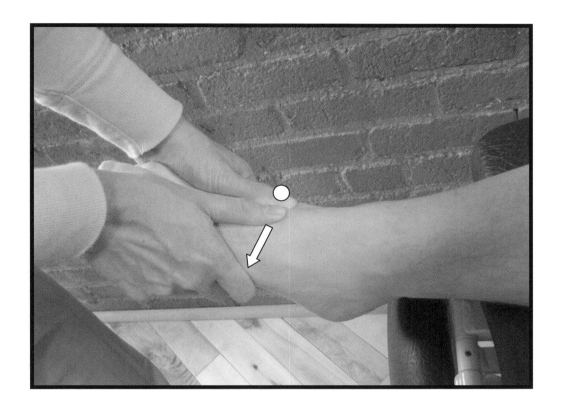

Technique described for the right medial intercuneiform joint

Patient: Supine lying with foot off edge of bed

Therapist: Standing at the end of the bed. Stabilize the middle cuneiform with your left hand. Grasp the medial cuneiform with your right index finger and thumb.

Action: Apply a plantar force to the medial cuneiform. Note the range of motion, end feel and reproduction of symptoms. Repeat the technique for a dorsal glide of the lateral cuneiform on the middle cuneiform.

The Mid Foot
Stability Testing

Stability Tests

Ligament Stress Tests

Stability Test
Midtarsal Traction and Compression

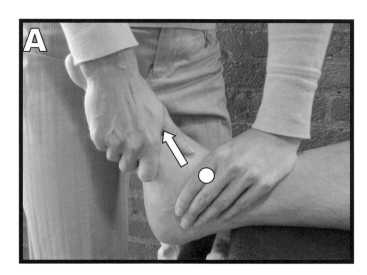 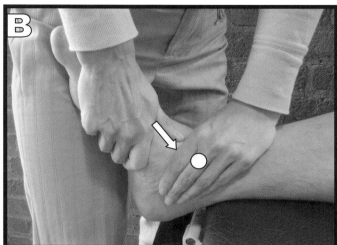

Technique described for the right talonavicular joint

Patient: Supine lying with foot off edge of bed

Therapist: Stand at the end of the bed. Stabilize the talus with your left hand. Grasp the navicular with your right index finger and thumb.

Action: Apply a traction (A) or compression (B) force to the navicular. Note the end feel and reproduction of symptoms. Repeat the technique for the calcaneocuboid, cuneonavicular and cuneocuboid joints.

Stability Test
Talonavicular Dorsal Translation

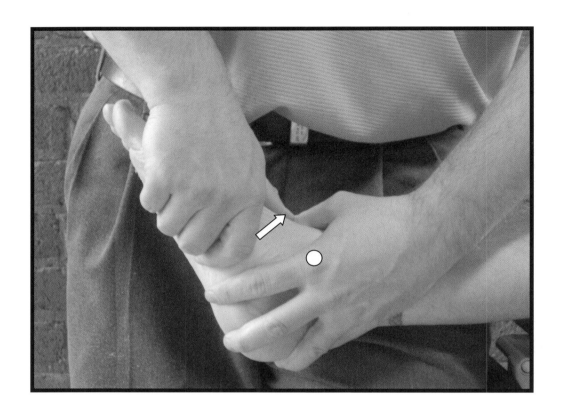

Technique described for the right talonavicular joint

Patient: Supine lying with foot off edge of bed

Therapist: Standing at the end of the bed. Stabilize the head of the talus with your left hand. Grasp the navicular with your right index finger and thumb.

Action: Apply a dorsal translation force to the navicular. Note the end feel and reproduction of symptoms.

Stability Test
Talonavicular Plantar Translation

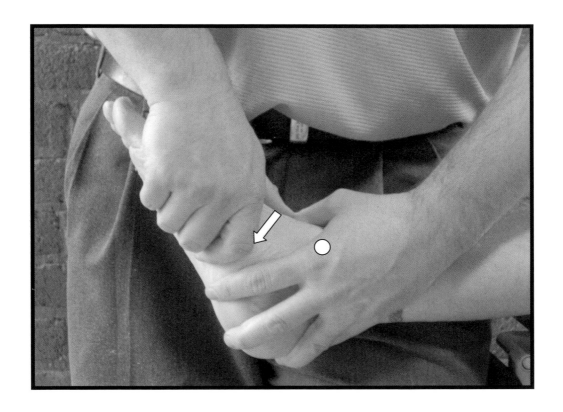

Technique described for the right talonavicular joint

Patient: Supine lying with foot off edge of bed

Therapist: Standing at the end of the bed. Stabilize the head of the talus with your left hand. Grasp the navicular with your right hand.

Action: Apply a plantar translation force to the navicular. Note the end feel and reproduction of symptoms.

Stability Test
Calcaneocuboid Dorsal Translation

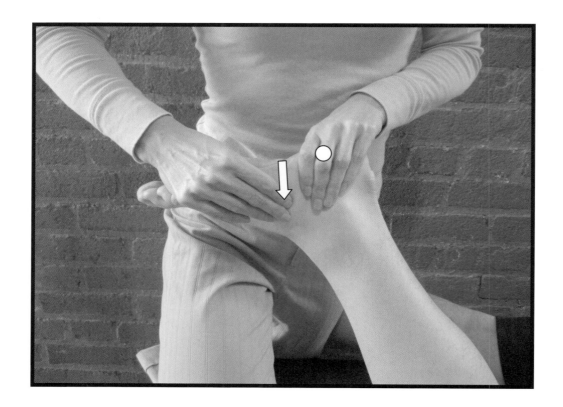

Technique described for the right calcaneocuboid joint

Patient: Prone lying with the knee flexed

Therapist: Standing at the end of the bed. Stabilize the calcaneus with your left hand.
Grasp the cuboid with your right index finger and thumb.

Action: Apply a dorsal translation force to the cuboid. Note the end feel and
reproduction of symptoms.

Stability Test
Calcaneocuboid Plantar Translation

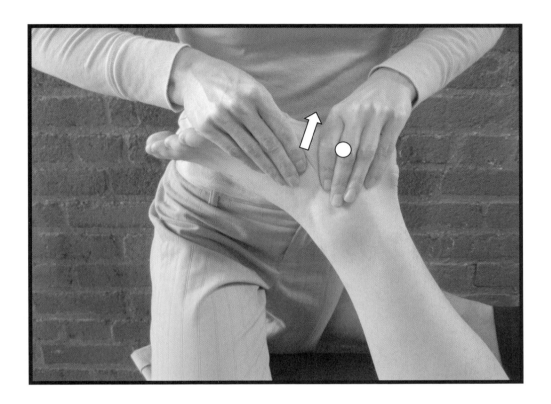

Technique described for the right calcaneocuboid joint

Patient: Prone lying with the knee flexed

Therapist: Standing at the end of the bed. Stabilize the calcaneus with your left hand. Grasp the cuboid with your right index finger and thumb.

Action: Apply a plantar translation force to the cuboid. Note the end feel and reproduction of symptoms.

Stability Test
Cuneonavicluar, Cuneocuboid, and Intercuneiform Dorsal Translation

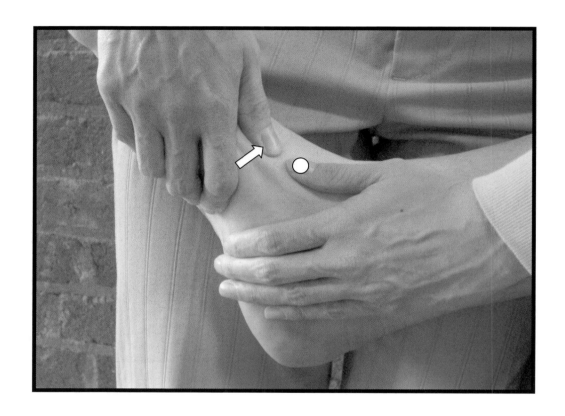

Technique described for the right medial cuneonavicular joint

Patient: Supine lying with foot off edge of bed

Therapist: Standing at the end of the bed. Stabilize the navicular with your left hand. Grasp the medial cuneiform with your right index finger and thumb.

Action: Apply a dorsal translation force to the medial cuneiform. Note the end feel and reproduction of symptoms. Repeat this technique for the cuneocuboid and intercuneiform joints.

Stability Test
Cuneonavicular, Cuneocuboid, and Intercuneiform Plantar Translation

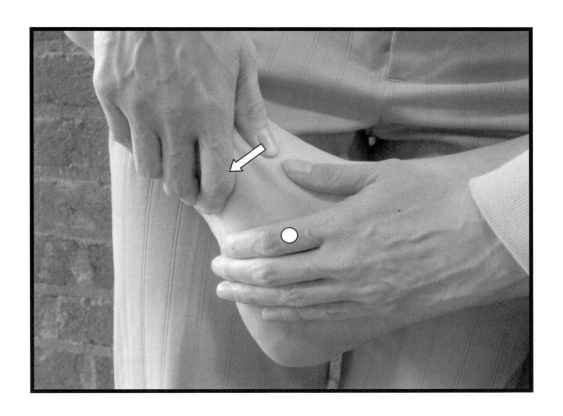

Technique described for the right medial cuneonavicular joint

Patient: Supine lying with foot off edge of bed

Therapist: Standing at the end of the bed. Stabilize the navicular with your left hand. Grasp the medial cuneiform with your right index finger and thumb.

Action: Apply a plantar translation force to the medial cuneiform. Note the end feel and reproduction of symptoms. Repeat this technique for the cuneocuboid and intercuneiform joints.

Ligament Stress Test
Dorsal Calcaneocuboid Ligament

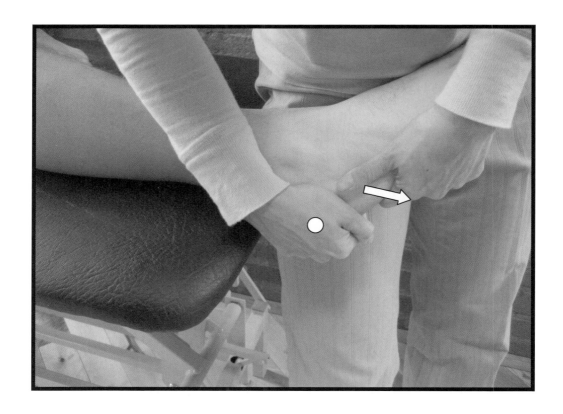

Technique described for the right calcaneocuboid joint

Patient: Supine lying with foot off edge of bed

Therapist: Standing at the end of the bed. Stabilize the calcaneus in pronation with your right hand. Grasp the cuboid with your left index finger and thumb .

Action: Invert and adduct the cuboid with your left hand. This will stress the dorsal calcaneocuboid ligament. Note the end feel and reproduction of symptoms.

Ligament Stress Test
Dorsal Talonavicular Ligament

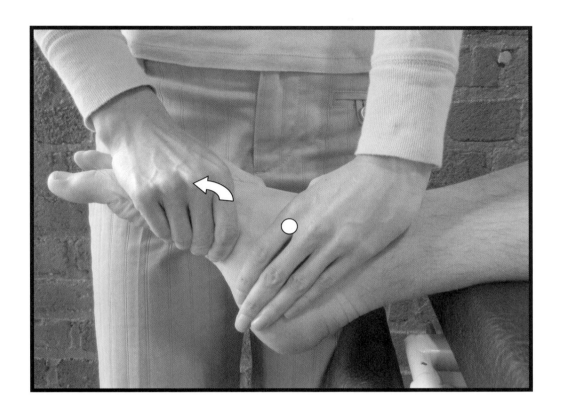

Technique described for the right talonavicular joint

Patient: Supine lying with foot off edge of bed

Therapist: Standing at the end of the bed. Stabilize the talus with your left hand.
Grasp the navicular with your right hand.

Action: Plantarflex the navicular and gap the dorsal aspect of the talonavicular joint.
This will stress the dorsal talonavicular ligament. Note the end feel and reproduction of
symptoms.

Ligament Stress Test
Plantar Calcaneocuboid Ligament

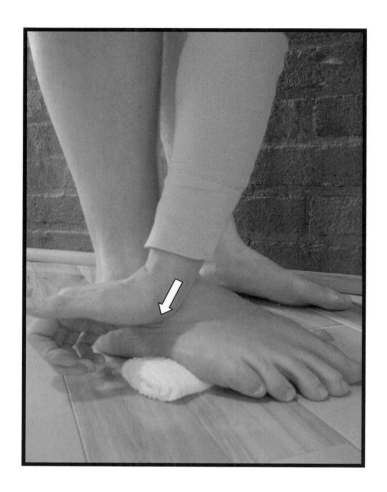

Technique described for the right calcaneocuboid joint

Patient: Standing with a rolled face cloth under the base of the fifth metatarsal

Therapist: Crouched facing the patient. Place the pisiform of your right hand on the dorsal aspect the cuboid. The floor will stabilize the calcaneus.

Action: Apply a plantar force to the cuboid. This will stress the plantar calcaneocuboid ligament. Note the end feel and reproduction of symptoms.

Ligament Stress Test

Plantar Calcaneonavicular Ligament (Spring Ligament)

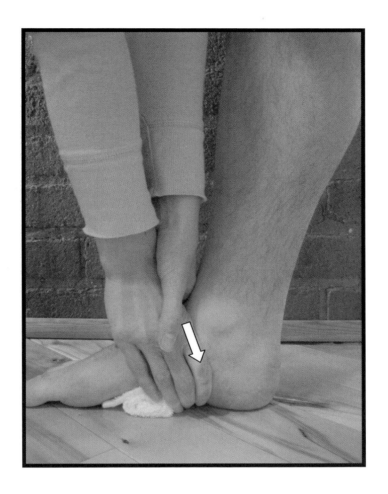

Technique described for the right talonavicular joint

Patient: Standing with a rolled face cloth under the navicular

Therapist: Crouched facing the patient. Place the metacarpalphalangeal border of your right index finger on the head of the talus. Reinforce your right hand with your left hand. The floor will stabilize the calcaneus.

Action: Apply a plantar force to the head of the talus. This will stress the plantar calcaneonavicular ligament (spring ligament). Note the end feel and reproduction of symptoms.

Ligament Stress Test
Bifurcate Ligament - Calcaneocuboid Portion

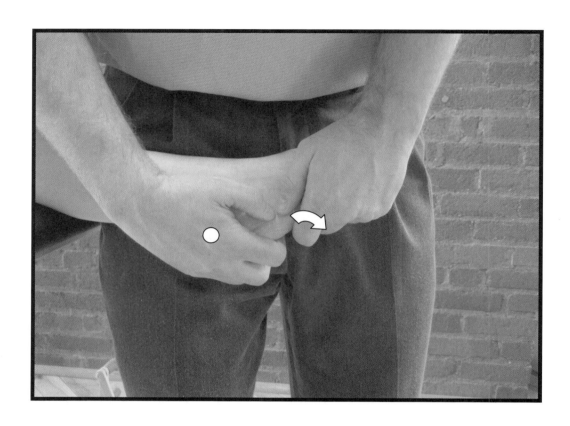

Technique described for the right calcaneocuboid joint

Patient: Supine lying with foot off edge of bed

Therapist: Standing at the end of the bed. Stabilize the calcaneus with your right hand. Grasp the cuboid with your left index finger and thumb .

Action: Plantarflex the cuboid and apply a varus force. This will stress the calcaneocuboid portion of he bifurcate ligament. Note the end feel and reproduction of symptoms.

Ligament Stress Test
Bifurcate Ligament – Calcaneonavicular Portion

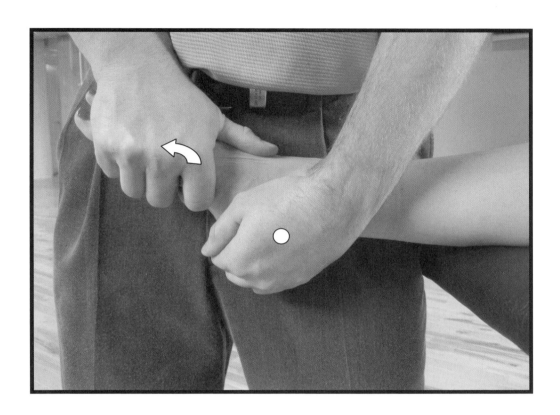

Technique described for the right midfoot

Patient: Supine lying with foot off edge of bed

Therapist: Standing at the end of the bed. Stabilize the calcaneus with your left hand. Grasp the navicular with your right index finger and thumb.

Action: Plantarflex the navicular and apply a valgus force. This will stress the calcaneonavicular portion of the bifurcate ligament. Note the end feel and reproduction of symptoms.

The Midfoot
Treatment Techniques

Passive Physiological Mobilization

Passive Accessory Mobilization

Treatment Technique
Passive Physiological Mobilization
Pronation (Dorsiflexion-Abduction-Eversion)

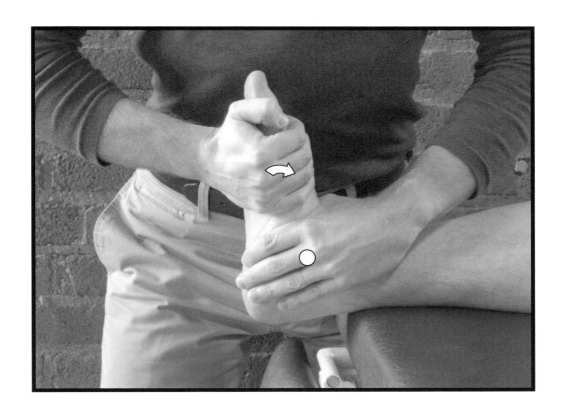

Technique described for the right midfoot

Indication: Restriction of pronation

Patient: Supine lying with foot off edge of bed

Therapist: Standing at the end of the bed. Stabilize the talus and calcaneus with your left hand. Grasp the sole of the foot with your right hand.

Action: Mobilize the patient's midfoot into pronation (dorsiflexion-abduction-eversion). This technique can be graded from 1 to 4.

Treatment Technique

Passive Physiological Mobilization
Supination (Plantarflexion-Adduction-Inversion)

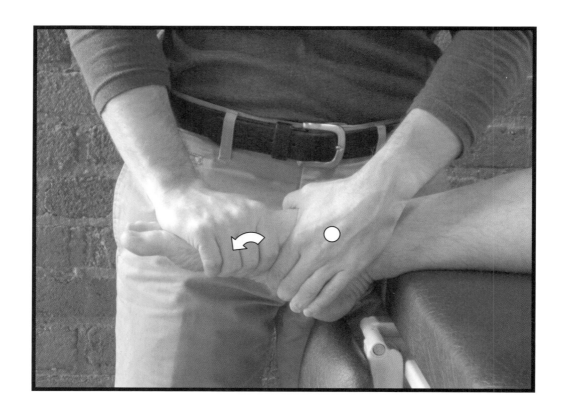

Technique described for the right midfoot

Indication: Restriction of supination in the midfoot

Patient: Supine lying with foot off edge of bed

Therapist: Standing at the end of the bed. Stabilize the talus and calcaneus with your left hand. Grasp the forefoot with your right hand.

Action: Mobilize the patient's midfoot into supination (plantarflexion-adduction-inversion). This technique can be graded from 1 to 4.

Treatment Technique
Talonavicular Dorsal Glide

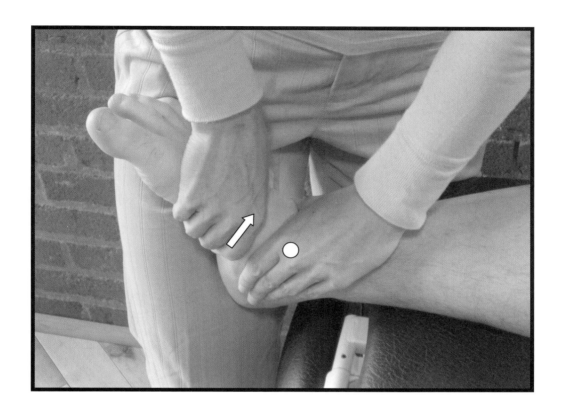

Technique described for the right talonavicular joint

Indication: Articular restriction of pronation

Patient: Supine lying with foot off edge of bed

Therapist: Standing at the end of the bed. Stabilize the head of the talus with your left hand. Grasp the navicular with your right hand.

Action: Apply a dorsal glide to the navicular allowing the conjunct external rotation to occur. This technique can be graded from 1 to 4

Treatment Technique
Talonavicular Plantar Glide

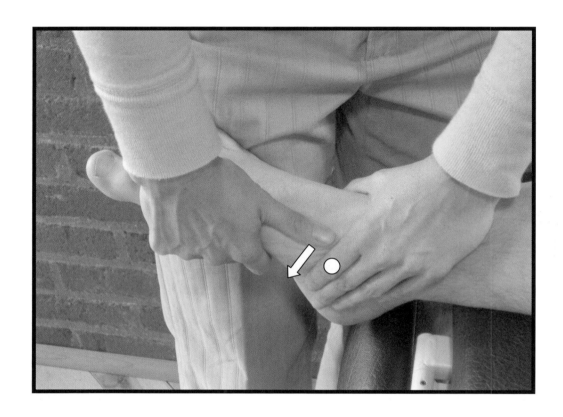

Technique described for the right talonavicular joint

Indication: Articular restriction of supination

Patient: Supine lying with foot off edge of bed

Therapist: Standing at the end of the bed. Stabilize the head of the talus with your left hand. Grasp the navicular with your right index finger and thumb.

Action: Apply a plantar glide to the navicular allowing the conjunct internal rotation to occur. This technique can be graded from 1 to 4.

Treatment Technique
Calcaneocuboid Dorsal Glide

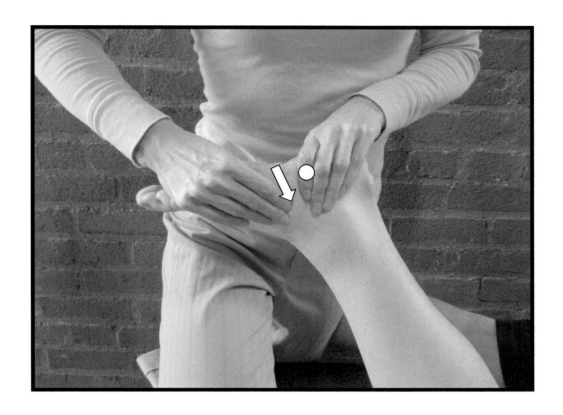

Technique described for the right calcaneocuboid joint

Indication: Articular restriction of pronation

Patient: Prone lying with the knee flexed

Therapist: Standing at the end of the bed. Stabilize the calcaneus with your left hand. Grasp the cuboid with your right index finger and thumb.

Action: Apply a dorsal glide to the cuboid allowing the conjunct internal rotation and abduction to occur. This technique can be graded from 1 to 4.

Treatment Technique
Calcaneocuboid Plantar Glide

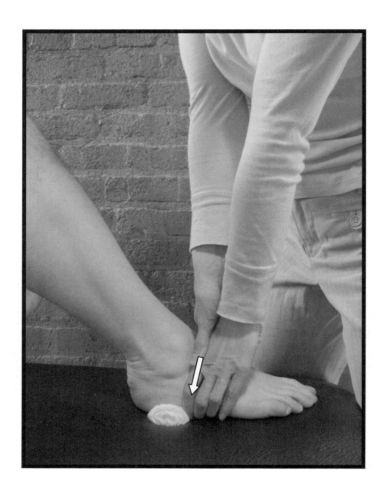

Technique described for the right calcaneocuboid joint

Indication: Articular restriction of supination

Patient: Crook lying with a rolled face cloth under the patient's calcaneus

Therapist: Standing at the end of the bed. Place your left second metacarpophalangeal joint over the dorsal aspect of the cuboid. Reinforce your left hand with your right hand.

Action: Apply a plantar glide to the cuboid allowing the conjunct external rotation and adduction to occur. This technique can be graded from 1 to 4.

Treatment Technique
Cuneonavicular Joint Dorsal Glide

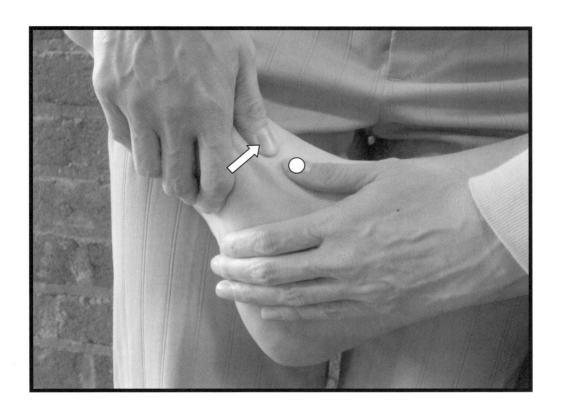

Technique described for the right cuneonavicular joint

Indication: Articular restriction of pronation

Patient: Supine lying with foot off edge of bed

Therapist: Standing at the end of the bed. Stabilize the navicular with your left hand. Grasp the medial cuneiform with your right index finger and thumb.

Action: Apply a dorsal glide to the medial cuneiform allowing the conjunct external rotation to occur. This technique can be graded from 1 to 4.

Treatment Technique
Cuneonavicular Joint Plantar Glide

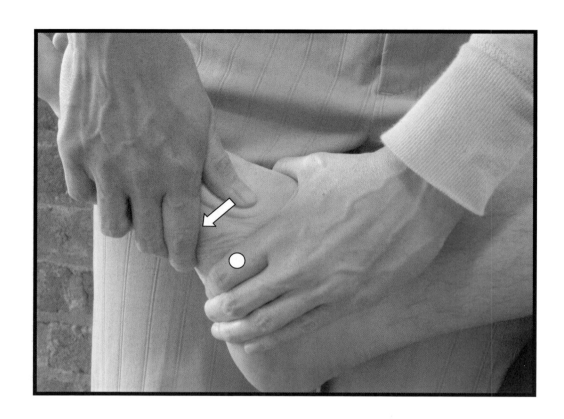

Technique described for the right cuneonavicular joint

Indication: Articular restriction of supination

Patient: Supine lying with foot off edge of bed

Therapist: Standing at the end of the bed. Stabilize the navicular with your left hand. Grasp the medial cuneiform with your right index finger and thumb.

Action: Apply a plantar glide to the medial cuneiform allowing the conjunct internal rotation to occur. This technique can be graded from 1 to 4.

Treatment Technique
Cuneocuboid Joint Dorsal Glide

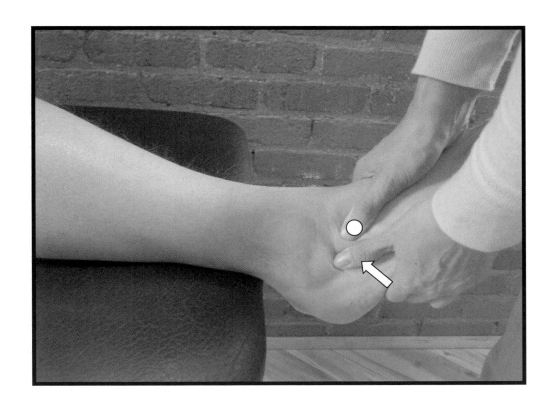

Technique described for the right cuneocuboid joint

Indication: Articular restriction of pronation

Patient: Supine lying with foot off edge of bed

Therapist: Standing at the end of the bed. Stabilize the lateral cuneiform with your right hand. Grasp the cuboid with your left index finger and thumb.

Action: Apply a dorsal glide to the cuboid. This technique can be graded from 1 to 4.

Treatment Technique
Cuneocuboid Joint Plantar Glide

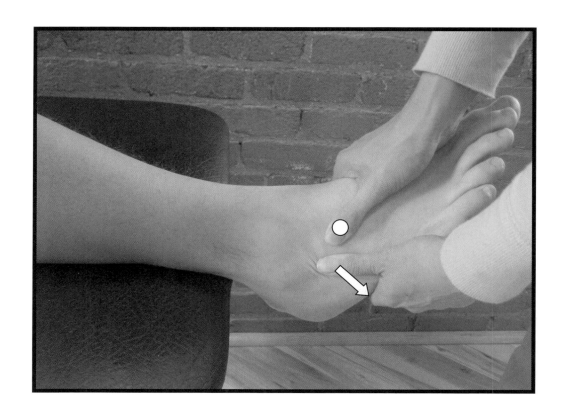

Technique described for the right cuneocuboid joint

Indication: Restriction of supination

Patient: Supine lying with foot off edge of bed

Therapist: Standing at the end of the bed. Stabilize the lateral cuneiform with your right hand. Grasp the cuboid with your left index finger and thumb.

Action: Apply a plantar glide to the cuboid. This technique can be graded from 1 to 4.

Treatment Technique
Intercuneiform Joint Dorsal Glide

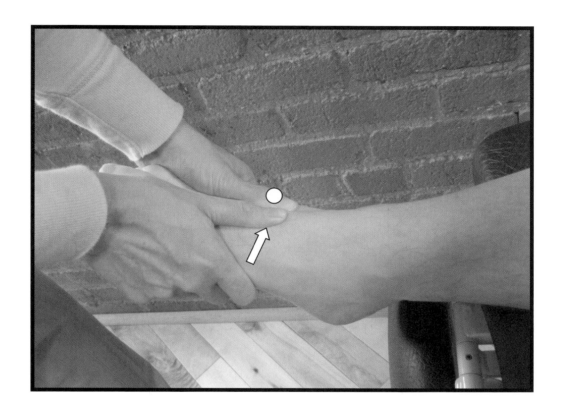

Technique described for the right medial intercuneiform joint

Indication: Articular restriction of pronation at the medial intercuneiform joint or supination at the lateral intercuneiform joint

Patient: Supine lying with foot off edge of bed

Therapist: Standing at the end of the bed. Stabilize the middle cuneiform with your left hand. Grasp the medial cuneiform with your right index finger and thumb.

Action: Apply a dorsal glide to the medial cuneiform. This technique can be graded from 1 to 4. This technique can be applied to the lateral cuneiform moving on the middle cuneiform.

Treatment Technique
Intercuneiform Joint Plantar Glide

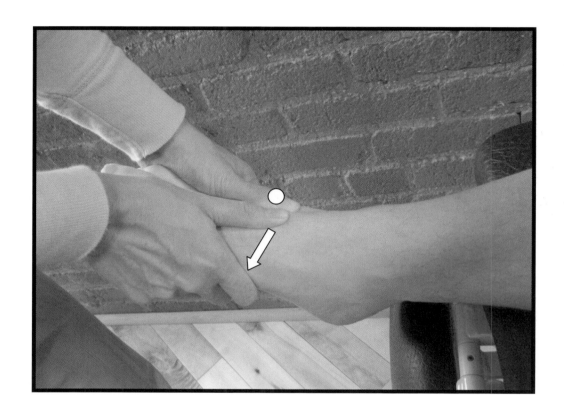

Technique described for the right medial intercuneiform joint

Indication: Articular restriction of supination at the medial intercuneiform joint or pronation at the lateral intercuneiform joint

Patient: Supine lying with foot off edge of bed

Therapist: Standing at the end of the bed. Stabilize the middle cuneiform with your left hand. Grasp the medial cuneiform with your right index finger and thumb.

Action: Apply a plantar glide to the medial cuneiform. This technique can be graded from 1 to 4. This technique can be applied to the lateral cuneiform moving on the middle cuneiform.

The Forefoot

The Forefoot
Active and Passive Movement Testing

Weight Bearing Range of Motion
Pronation
(Body Twist and Squat)

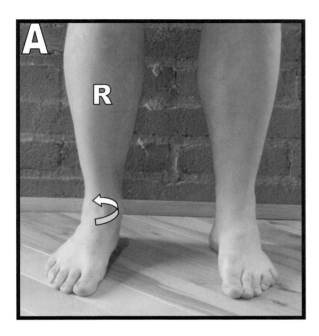 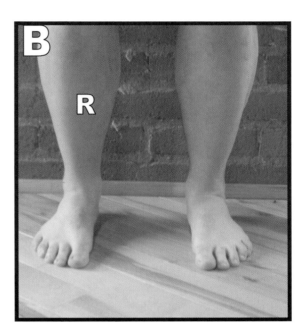

Technique described for the right forefoot

Patient: Standing with feet pointing straight ahead

Therapist: Crouched facing the patient

Action: Instruct the patient to twist to the left (A). Instruct the patient to partially squat while keeping their heels on the ground (B). Observe the range of motion in the forefoot. These two movements will cause the right forefoot to pronate and fan.

Weight Bearing Range of Motion
Supination
(Body Twist and Up on Toes)

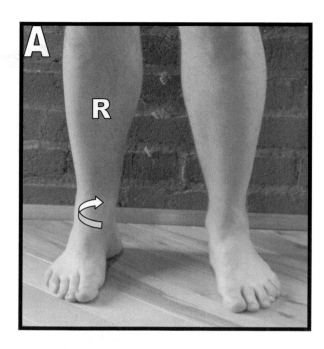 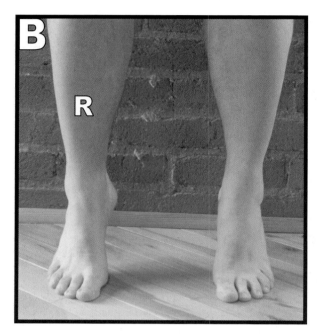

Technique described for the right forefoot

Patient: Standing with feet pointing straight ahead

Therapist: Crouched facing the patient

Action: Instruct the patient to twist to the right (A). Instruct the patient to raise up on their toes (B). Observe the range of motion in the forefoot. These two movements will cause the right forefoot to supinate and fold.

Passive Range of Motion
Dorsiflexion and Plantarflexion

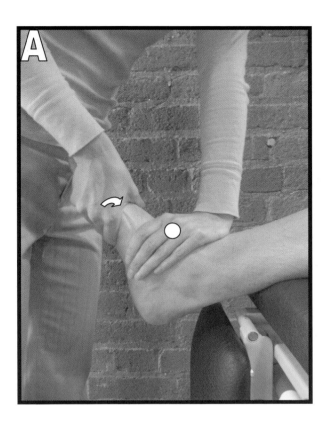 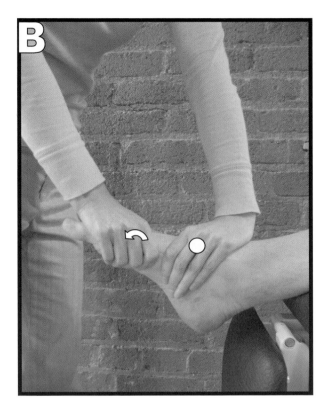

Technique described for the right forefoot

Patient: Supine lying with foot off edge of bed

Therapist: Standing at the end of the bed. Stabilize the midtarsal bones with your left hand. Grasp the metatarsal bases of the foot with your right hand.

Action: Passively dorsiflex (A) or plantarflex (B) the patient's forefoot. Note the range of motion, end feel and reproduction of symptoms.

Passive Range of Motion
Fanning and Folding

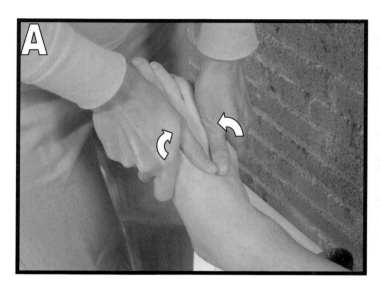 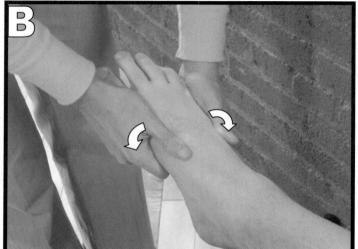

Technique described for the right forefoot

Patient: Supine lying with foot off edge of bed

Therapist: Standing at the end of the bed. Grasp the foot with both hands placing your thumbs along the midline.

Action: Passively fan (A) the patient's forefoot by moving the medial and lateral borders of the forefoot in a dorsal direction. Passively fold (B) the patient's forefoot by moving the medial and lateral borders of the forefoot in a plantar direction. Note the range of motion, end feel and reproduction of symptoms.

Passive Range of Motion
MTP and IP Flexion and Extension

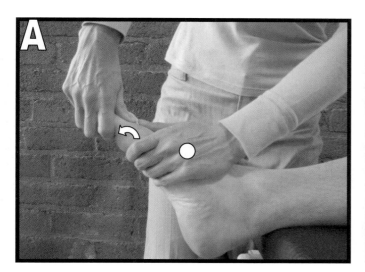 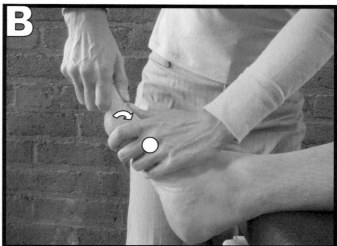

Technique described for the right first MTP joint

Patient: Supine lying with foot off edge of bed

Therapist: Standing at the end of the bed. Stabilize the first metatarsal with your left hand. Grasp the first proximal phalanx with your right index finger and thumb.

Action: Passively flex (A) or extend (B) the patient's first MTP joint. Note the range of motion, end feel and reproduction of symptoms. Repeat these techniques for the second to fifth MTP joints and the first to fifth IP joints.

Passive Range of Motion
MTP Abduction

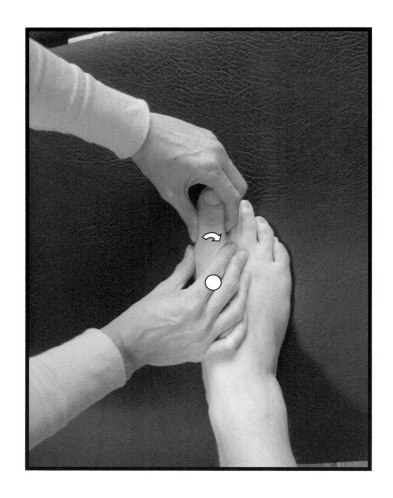

Technique described for the right first MTP joint

Patient: Crook lying with right foot flat on bed

Therapist: Standing at the end of the bed. Stabilize the first metatarsal with your right hand. Grasp the first proximal phalanx with your left index finger and thumb.

Action: Passively abduct the patient's first MTP joint. Note the range of motion, end feel and reproduction of symptoms. Repeat this technique for the second to fifth MTP joints.

Passive Range of Motion
MTP Adduction

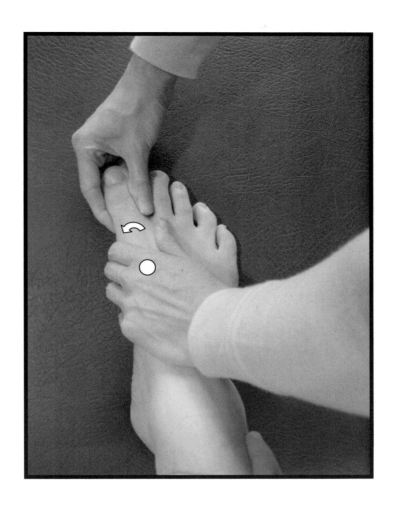

Technique described for the right first MTP joint

Patient: Crook lying with right foot flat on bed

Therapist: Standing at the end of the bed. Stabilize the first metatarsal with your left hand. Grasp the first proximal phalanx with your right index finger and thumb.

Action: Passively adduct the patient's right first MTP joint. Note the range of motion, end feel and reproduction of symptoms. Repeat this technique for the second to fifth MTP joints.

Passive Accessory Motion
TMT Dorsal Glide

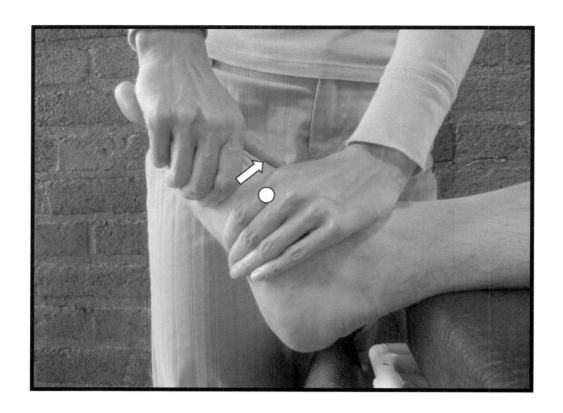

Technique described for the right first TMT joint

Patient: Supine lying with foot off edge of bed

Therapist: Standing at the end of the bed. Stabilize the medial cuneiform with your left hand. Grasp the first metatarsal with your right index finger and thumb.

Action: Apply a dorsal force to the base of the first metatarsal allowing the conjunct external rotation occur. Note the range of motion, end feel and reproduction of symptoms. Repeat the technique for the second to fifth TMT joints.

Passive Accessory Motion
TMT Plantar Glide

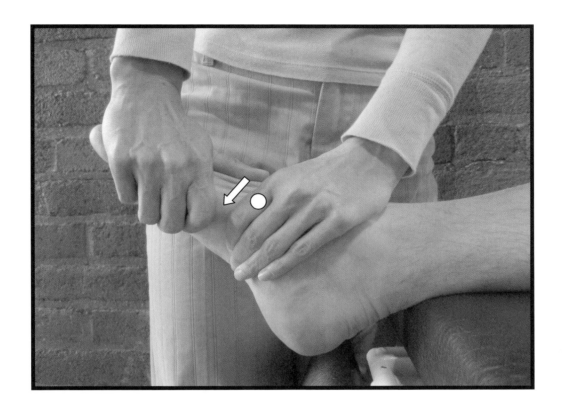

Technique described for the right first TMT Joint

Patient: Supine lying with foot off edge of bed

Therapist: Standing at the end of the bed. Stabilize the medial cuneiform with your left hand. Grasp the first metatarsal with your right index finger and thumb.

Action: Apply a plantar force to the base of the first metatarsal allowing the conjunct internal rotation to occur. Note the range of motion, end feel and reproduction of symptoms. Repeat the technique for the second to fifth TMT joints.

Passive Accessory Motion
Intermetatarsal Dorsal and Plantar Glide

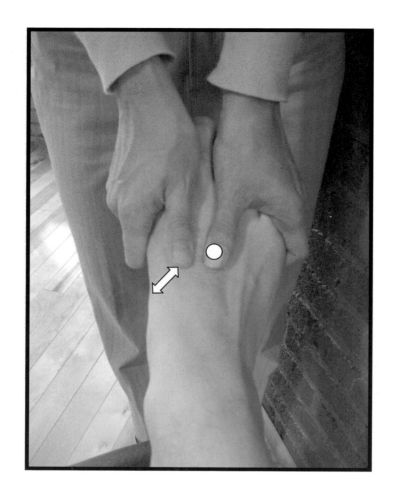

Technique described for the right first intermetatarsal joint

Patient: Supine lying with foot off edge of bed

Therapist: Standing at the end of the bed. Stabilize the second metatarsal with your left hand. Grasp the first metatarsal with your right index finger and thumb.

Action: Apply a dorsal or plantar force to the first metatarsal. Note the range of motion, end feel and reproduction of symptoms. Repeat the technique for the other intermetatarsal joints.

Passive Accessory Motion
MTP and IP Dorsal and Plantar Glide

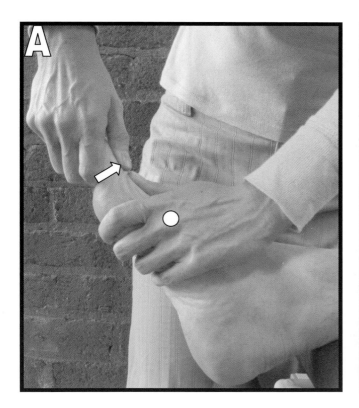
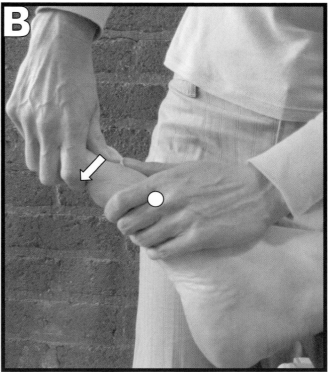

Technique described for the right first MTP Joint

Patient: Supine lying with foot off edge of bed

Therapist: Standing at the end of the bed. Stabilize the first metatarsal with your left hand. Grasp the first proximal phalanx with your right index finger and thumb.

Action: Apply a dorsal (A) or plantar (B) force to the proximal phalanx. Note the range of motion, end feel and reproduction of symptoms. Repeat this technique for the second to fifth MTP joints and the first to fifth IP joints.

Passive Accessory Motion
MTP Medial Glide

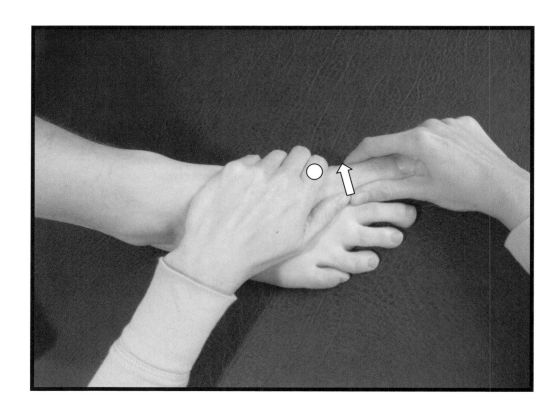

Technique described for the right first MTP joint

Patient: Crook lying with right foot flat on bed

Therapist: Standing at the end of the bed. Stabilize the first metatarsal with your left hand. Grasp the first proximal phalanx with your right index finger and thumb.

Action: Apply a medial force to the proximal phalanax. Note the range of motion, end feel and reproduction of symptoms. Repeat this technique for the second to fifth MTP joints.

Passive Accessory Motion
MTP Lateral Glide

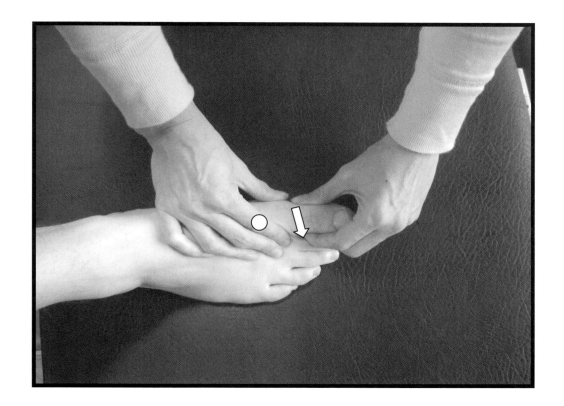

Technique described for the right first MTP Joint

Patient: Crook lying with right foot flat on bed

Therapist: Standing at the end of the bed. Stabilize the first metatarsal with your right hand. Grasp the first proximal phalanx with your left index finger and thumb.

Action: Apply a lateral force to the proximal phalanax. Note the range of motion, end feel and reproduction of symptoms. Repeat this technique for the second to fifth MTP joints.

The Forefoot
Stability Testing

Passive Stability Test
TMT Traction and Compression

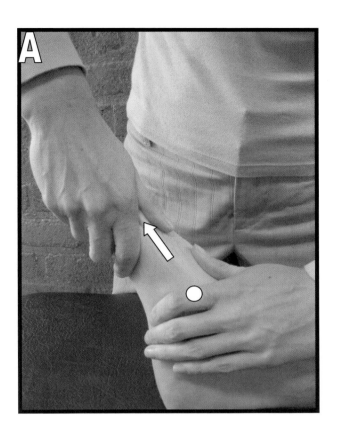 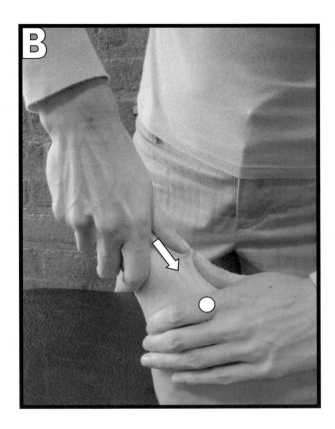

Technique described for the right first TMT Joint

Patient: Supine Lying

Therapist: Standing at the end of the bed. Stabilize the medial cuneiform with your left hand. Grasp the first metatarsal with your right index finger and thumb.

Action: Apply a traction (A) or compression (B) force to the base of the first metatarsal. Note the end feel and reproduction of symptoms. Repeat the technique for the second to fifth TMT joints.

Passive Stability Test
TMT Dorsal Translation

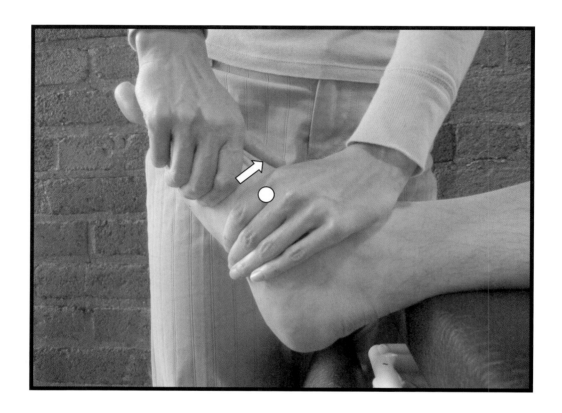

Technique described for the right first TMT joint

Patient: Supine lying with foot off edge of bed

Therapist: Standing at the end of the bed. Stabilize the medial cuneiform with your left hand. Grasp the first metatarsal with your right index finger and thumb.

Action: Apply a dorsal translation force to the first metatarsal. Note the end feel and reproduction of symptoms. Repeat the technique for the second to fifth TMT joints.

Passive Stability Test
TMT Plantar Translation

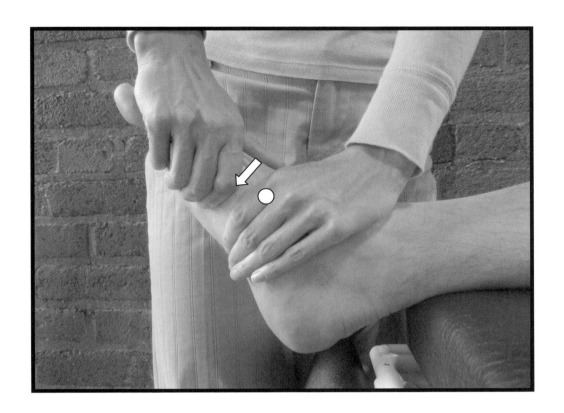

Technique described for the right first TMT Joint

Patient: Supine lying with foot off edge of bed

Therapist: Standing at the end of the bed. Stabilize the medial cuneiform with your left hand. Grasp the first metatarsal with your right index finger and thumb.

Action: Apply a plantar translation force to the first metatarsal. Note the end feel and reproduction of symptoms. Repeat the technique for the second to fifth TMT joints.

Passive Stability Test
Intermetatarsal Dorsal and Plantar Translation

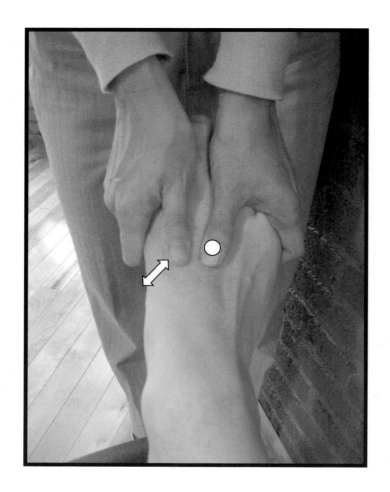

Technique described for the right first intermetatarsal joint

Patient: Supine lying with foot off edge of bed

Therapist: Standing at the end of the bed. Stabilize the second metatarsal with your left hand. Grasp the first metatarsal with your right hand.

Action: Apply a dorsal or plantar translation force to the first metatarsal. Note the end feel and reproduction of symptoms. Repeat the technique for the other intermetatarsal joints.

Passive Stability Test
MTP and IP Traction and Compression

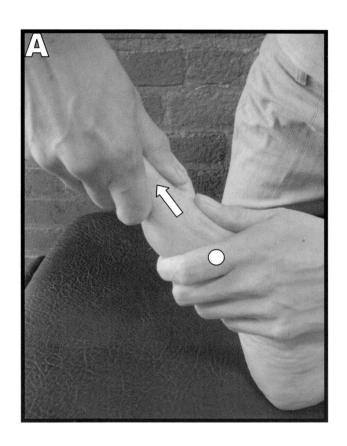 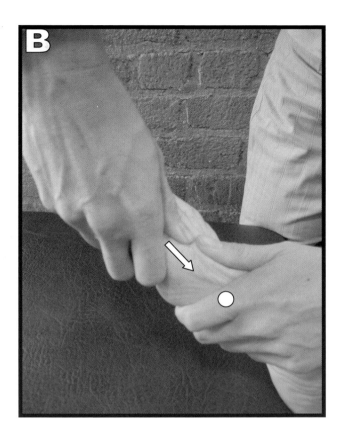

Technique described for the right first MTP joint

Patient: Supine lying

Therapist: Standing at the side of the bed. Stabilize the first metatarsal with your left index finger and thumb. Grasp the first proximal phalanax with your right index finger and thumb.

Action: Apply a traction (A) or compression (B) force to the proximal phalanx. Note the end feel and reproduction of symptoms. Repeat this technique for the second to fifth MTP joints and the first to fifth IP joints.

Passive Stability Test
MTP and IP Dorsal and Plantar Translation

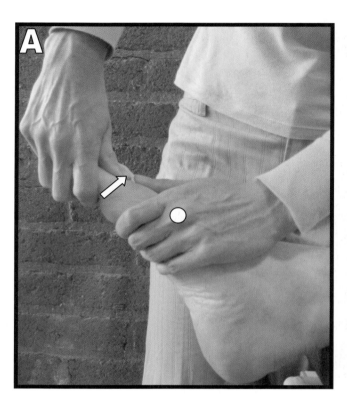 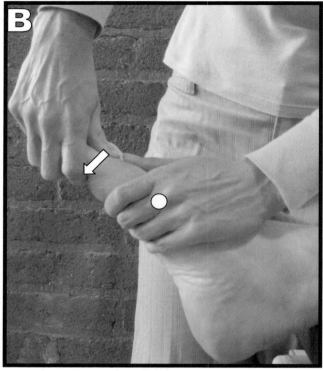

Technique described for the right first MTP joint

Patient: Supine lying with foot off edge of bed

Therapist: Standing at the end of the bed. Stabilize the first metatarsal with your left hand. Grasp the first proximal phalanx with your right index finger and thumb.

Action: Apply a dorsal (A) or a plantar (B) translation force to the proximal phalanx. Note the end feel and reproduction of symptoms. Repeat these techniques for the second to fifth MTP joints and the first to fifth IP joints.

Passive Stability Test
MTP and IP Valgus Stress

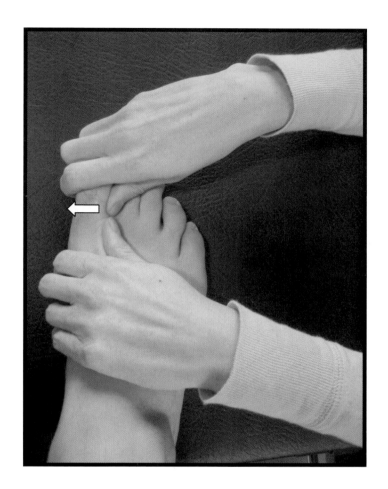

Technique described for the right first MTP joint

Patient: Crook lying with foot flat on bed

Therapist: Standing at the end of the bed. Stabilize the first metatarsal with your left index finger and thumb. Grasp the first proximal phalanx with your right index finger and thumb.

Action: Apply a valgus force to the first MTP joint. Note the end feel and reproduction of symptoms. Repeat this technique for the second to fifth MTP joints and first to fifth IP joints.

Passive Stability Test
MTP and IP Varus Stress

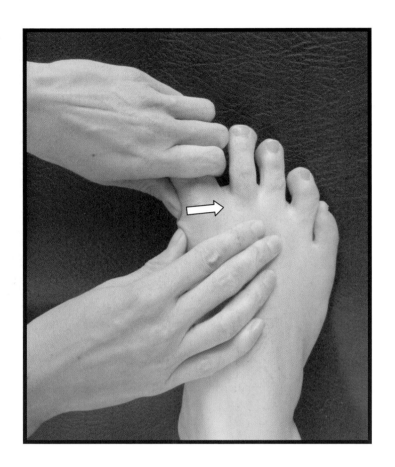

Technique described for the right first MTP joint

Patient: Crook lying with foot flat on bed

Therapist: Standing at the end of the bed. Stabilize the first metatarsal with your right index finger and thumb. Grasp the first proximal phalanx with your left index finger and thumb.

Action: Apply a varus force to the first MTP joint. Note the end feel and reproduction of symptoms. Repeat this technique for the second to fifth MTP joints and the first to fifth IP joints.

The Forefoot
Treatment Techniques

Passive Physiological Mobilization

Passive Accessory Mobilization

Treatment Technique
Passive Physiological Mobilization
Forefoot Dorsiflexion and Plantarflexion

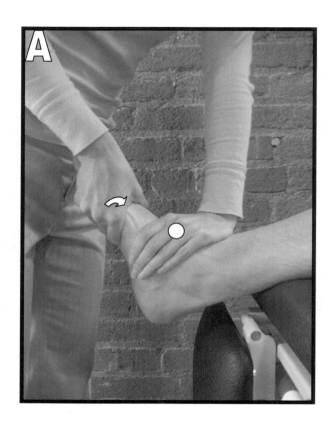 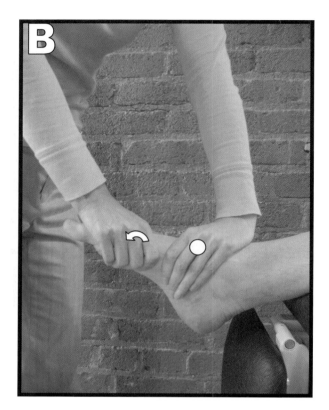

Technique described for the right forefoot

Indication: Restriction of dorsiflexion or plantarflexion in the forefoot

Patient: Supine lying with foot off edge of bed

Therapist: Standing at the end of the bed. Stabilize the midtarsal bones with your left hand. Grasp the metatarsal bases of the foot with your right hand.

Action: Mobilize the patient's forefoot through dorsiflexion (A) or plantarflexion (B). This technique can be graded from 1 to 4.

Treatment Technique
Passive Physiological Mobilization
Forefoot Fanning and Folding

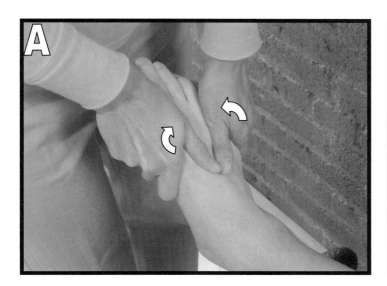
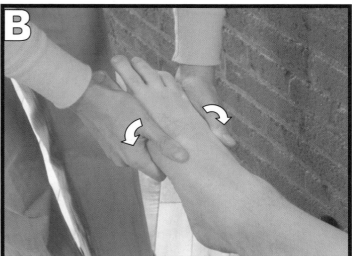

Technique described for the right forefoot

Indication: Restriction of fanning or folding in the forefoot

Patient: Supine lying with foot off edge of bed

Therapist: Standing at the end of the bed. Grasp the foot with both hands placing your thumbs along the midline.

Action: Mobilize the forefoot into fanning (A) by moving the medial and lateral borders of the forefoot in a dorsal direction. Mobilize the forefoot into folding (B) by moving the medial and lateral borders of the forefoot in a plantar direction. This technique can be graded from 1 to 4.

Treatment Technique
Passive Physiological Mobilization
MTP and IP Flexion and Extension

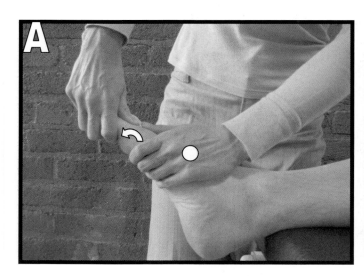 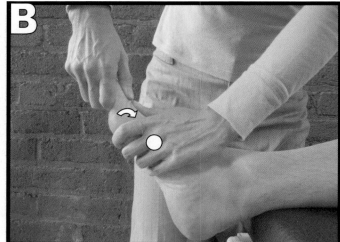

Technique described for the right first MTP joint

Indication: Restriction of flexion or extension of the first MTP joint

Patient: Supine lying with foot off edge of bed

Therapist: Standing at the end of the bed. Stabilize the first metatarsal with your left hand. Grasp the first proximal phalanx with your right index finger and thumb.

Action: Mobilize the first MTP joint into flexion (A) or extension (B). This technique can be graded from 1 to 4. This technique can be used for the second to fifth MTP joints and the first to fifth IP joints.

Treatment Technique
Passive Physiological Mobilization
MTP Abduction

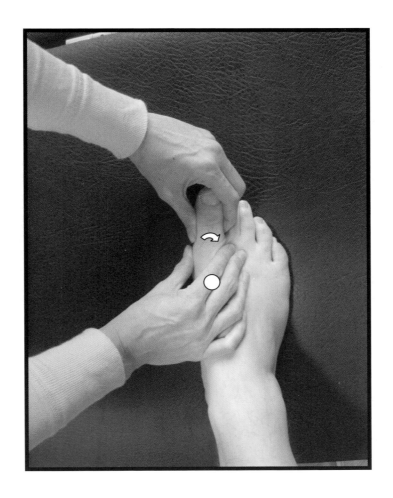

Technique described for the right first MTP joint

Indication: Restriction of abduction of the first MTP joint

Patient: Crook lying with right foot flat on bed

Therapist: Standing at the end of the bed. Stabilize the first metatarsal with your right hand. Grasp the first proximal phalanx with your left index finger and thumb.

Action: Mobilize the patient's first MTP joint into abduction. This technique can be graded from 1 to 4. This technique can be used for the second to fifth MTP joints.

Treatment Technique
Passive Physiological Mobilization
MTP Adduction

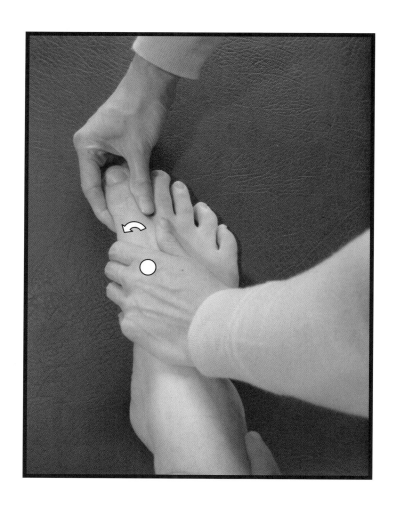

Technique described for the right first MTP joint

Indication: Restriction of adduction of the first MTP joint

Patient: Crook lying with right foot flat on bed

Therapist: Standing at the end of the bed. Stabilize the first metatarsal with your left hand. Grasp the first proximal phalanx with your right index finger and thumb.

Action: Mobilize the patient's first MTP joint into adduction. This technique can be graded from 1 to 4. This technique can be used for the second to fifth MTP joints.

Treatment Technique
TMT Traction

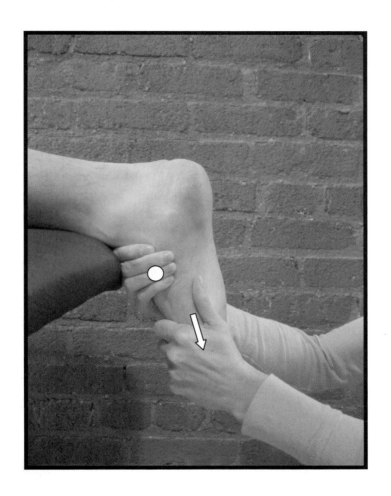

Technique described for the right first TMT joint

Indication: Articular restriction of the first TMT joint

Patient: Prone lying with foot off edge of bed

Therapist: Crouching at the end of the bed. Stabilize the medial cuneiform with your right hand. Grasp the first metatarsal with your left index finger and thumb.

Action: Apply a traction force to the first metatarsal. This technique can be graded form 1 to 4. This technique can be used for the second to fifth TMT joints.

Treatment Technique
TMT Dorsal Glide
First to Third TMT joints

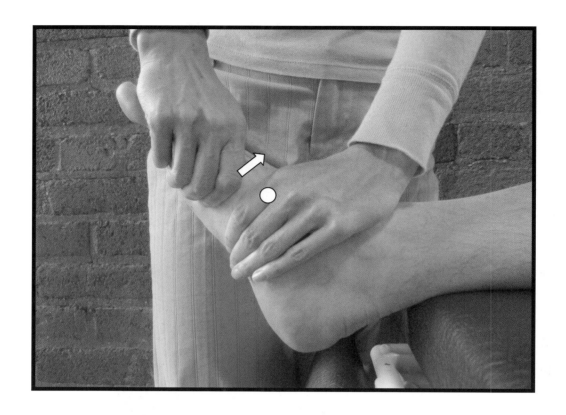

Technique described for the right first TMT joint

Indication: Articular restriction of dorsiflexion of the first TMT joint

Patient: Supine lying with foot off edge of bed

Therapist: Standing at the end of the bed. Stabilize the medial cuneiform with your left hand. Grasp the first metatarsal with your right index finger and thumb.

Action: Apply a dorsal glide to the base of the first metatarsal allowing the conjunct external rotation to occur. This technique can be graded from 1 to 4. This technique can be used for the second and third TMT joint.

Treatment Technique
TMT Dorsal Glide
Fourth and Fifth TMT Joints

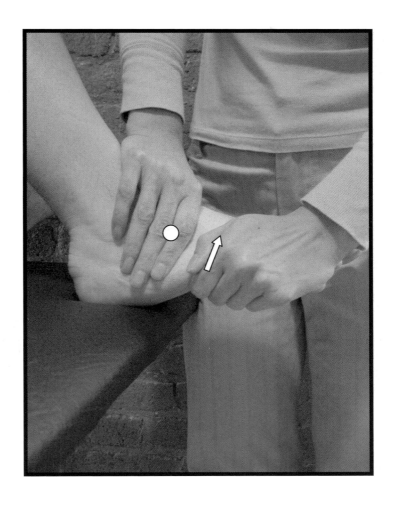

Technique described for the right fifth TMT joint

Indication: Articular restriction of plantarflexion of the fifth TMT joint

Patient: Supine lying with heel on edge of bed

Therapist: Standing at the end of the bed. Stabilize the cuboid with your right hand. Grasp the fifth metatarsal base with your left hand.

Action: Apply a dorsal glide to the fifth metatarsal. This technique can be graded from 1 to 4. This technique can be used for the fourth TMT joint.

Treatment Technique
TMT Plantar Glide
First to Third TMT joints

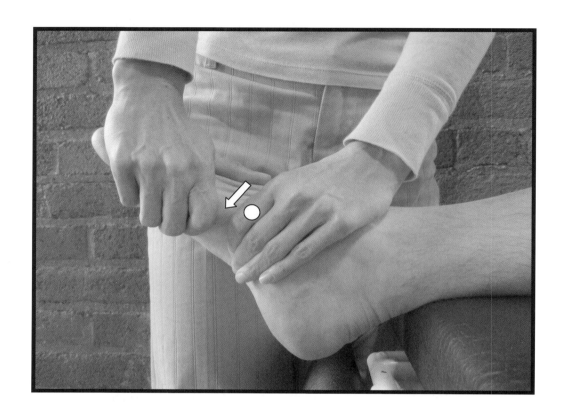

Technique described for the right first TMT joint

Indication: Articular restriction of plantarflexion of the first TMT joint

Patient: Supine lying with foot off edge of bed

Therapist: Standing at the end of the bed. Stabilize the medial cuneiform with your left hand. Grasp the first metatarsal with your right index finger and thumb.

Action: Apply a plantar glide to the base of the first metatarsal allowing the conjunct internal rotation to occur. This technique can be graded from 1 to 4. This technique can be used for the second and third TMT joint.

Treatment Technique
TMT Plantar Glide
Fourth and Fifth TMT Joints

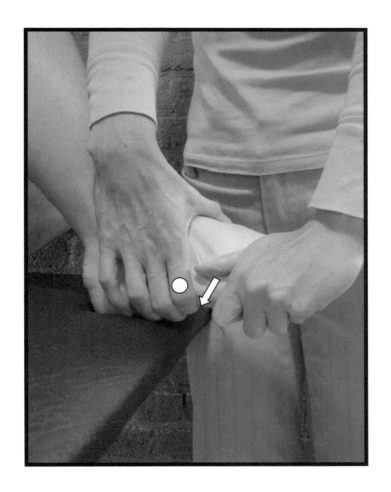

Technique described for the right fifth TMT joint

Indication: Articular restriction of dorsiflexion of the fifth TMT joint

Patient: Supine lying with heel on edge of bed

Therapist: Standing at the end of the bed. Stabilize the cuboid with your right hand. Grasp the fifth metatarsal base with your left index finger and thumb.

Action: Apply a plantar glide to the fifth metatarsal. This technique can be graded from 1 to 4. This technique can be used for the fourth TMT joint.

Treatment Technique
Intermetatarsal Joint Dorsal and Plantar Glide

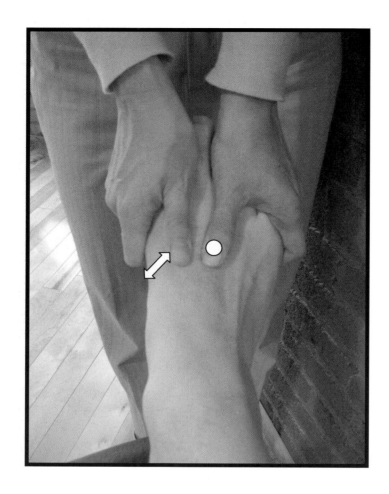

Technique described for the right first intermetatarsal joint

Indication: Articular restriction of folding or fanning

Patient: Supine lying with foot off edge of bed

Therapist: Standing at the end of the bed. Stabilize the second metatarsal with your left hand. Grasp the first metatarsal with your right hand.

Action: Apply a dorsal or plantar glide to the first metatarsal. This technique can be graded from 1 to 4. This technique can be used for the second to fourth intermetatarsal joints.

Treatment Technique
MTP and IP Traction

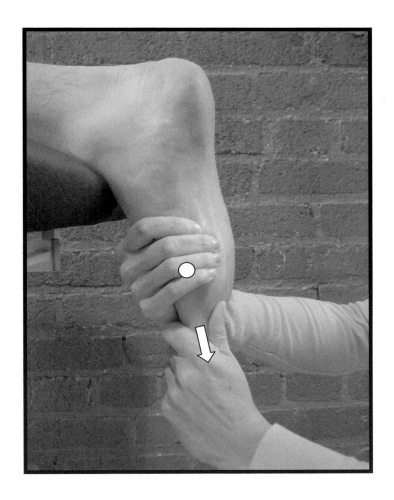

Technique described for the right first MTP joint

Indication: Articular restriction of the first MTP joint

Patient: Prone lying with foot off edge of bed

Therapist: Crouching at the end of the bed. Stabilize the first metatarsal with your right hand. Grasp the first proximal phalanx with your left index finger and thumb.

Action: Apply a traction force to the proximal phalanx. This technique can be graded form 1 to 4. This technique can be used for the second to fifth MTP joints and the first to fifth IP joints.

Treatment Technique
MTP and IP Dorsal and Plantar Glide

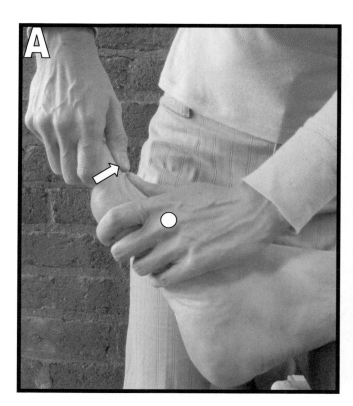 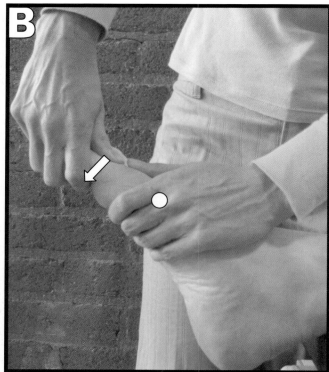

Technique described for the right first MTP joint

Indication: Articular restriction of flexion (A) or extension (B) at the first MTP joint

Patient: Supine lying with foot off edge of bed

Therapist: Standing at the end of the bed. Stabilize the first metatarsal with your left hand. Grasp the first proximal phalanx with your right index finger and thumb.

Action: Apply a dorsal glide to the proximal phalanx (A). Apply a plantar glide to the proximal phalanx (B). These techniques can be graded from 1 to 4. These techniques can be used for the second to fifth MTP joints and the first to fifth IP joints.

Treatment Technique
MTP Medial Glide

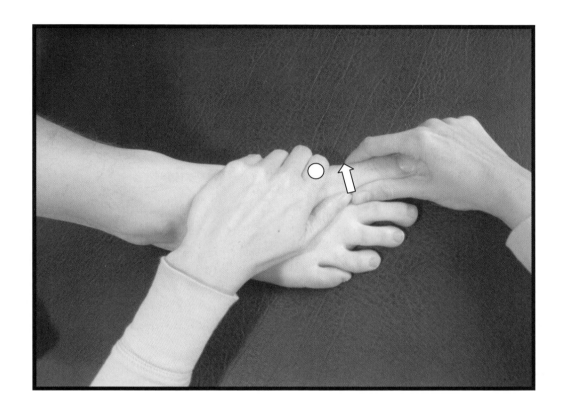

Technique described for the right first MTP joint

Indication: Articular restriction of adduction at the first MTP joint

Patient: Crook lying with right foot flat on bed

Therapist: Standing at the end of the bed. Stabilize the first metatarsal with your left hand. Grasp the first proximal phalanx with your right index finger and thumb.

Action: Apply a medial glide to the proximal phalanax. This technique can be graded from 1 to 4. This technique can be used for the second to fifth MTP joints.

Passive Accessory Motion
MTP Lateral Glide

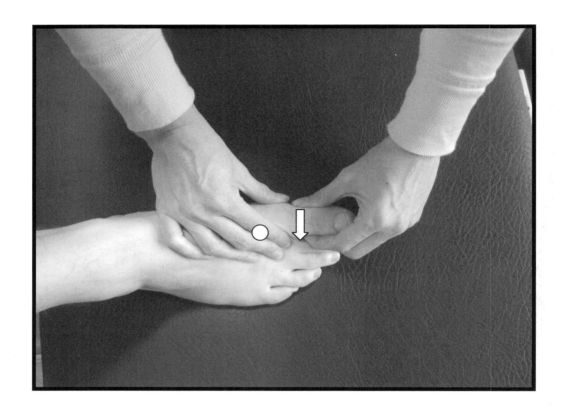

Technique described for the right first MTP Joint

Indication: Articular restriction of abduction at the first MTP joint

Patient: Crook lying with right foot flat on bed

Therapist: Standing at the end of the bed. Stabilize the first metatarsal with your right hand. Grasp the first proximal phalanx with your left index finger and thumb.

Action: Apply a lateral glide to the proximal phalanax. This technique can be graded from 1 to 4. This technique can be used for the second to fifth MTP joints.

Lower Quadrant Manipulations

Lower Quadrant Manipulations

Lower Quadrant Manipulations

Manipulation Technique
Loose Body Mobilization / Manipulation

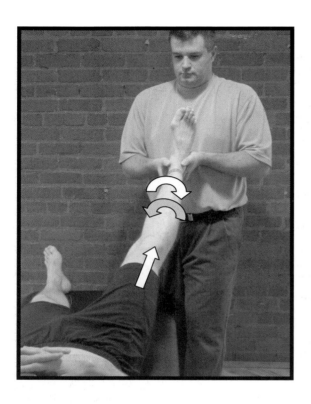 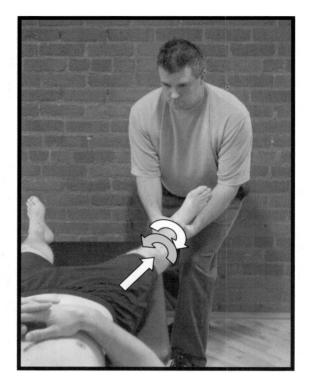

Technique described for the right hip

Indication: Loose body in the hip joint

Patient: Supine lying

Therapist: Standing at the end of the bed. Grasp the patients distal tibia and fibula with both hands.

Action: Position the patient's leg into 60 degrees of flexion. Passively assess which rotation of the leg is best tolerated by the patient. Apply a traction force while alternately flicking the patient's leg into the rotation which you found most comfortable and back to neutral while you bring the leg into extension.

Manipulation Technique
Tibio-Femoral Joint
Loose Body Mobilization / Manipulation

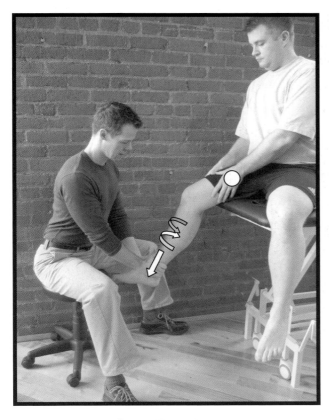

Start Position

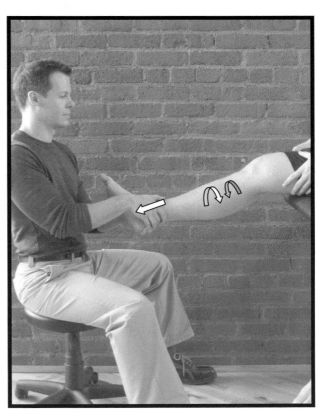

Finish Position

Technique described for the right knee with a extension block

Indication: Articular restriction of flexion or extension due to a loose body

Patient: Seated at the end of the bed while stabilizing the right femur with their hands

Therapist: Seated or kneeling at the foot of the bed. Grasp the distal tibia and fibula with both hands.

Action: Apply a traction force to the tibio-femoral joint. Rotate the tibia back and forth as you move the joint from flexion to extension. Maintain the distraction throughout the movement. This technique can be repeated for a flexion block by rotating the tibia back and forth as you move the joint from extension to flexion.

Manipulation Technique
Tibio-Femoral Joint
Lateral Glide of Tibia (Relative Technique)

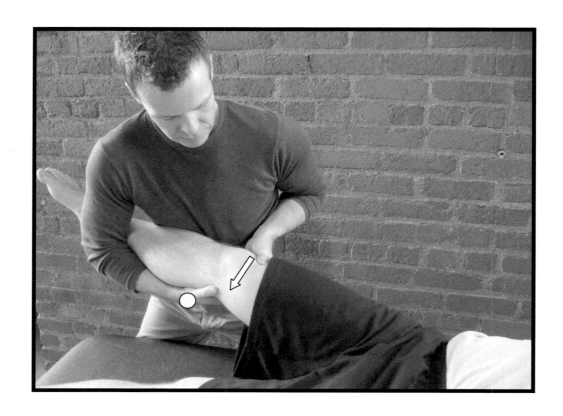

Technique described for the right tibio-femoral joint

Indication: Articular restriction of abduction

Patient: Supine with knee slightly flexed

Therapist: Standing at the side of bed with the patient's leg supported between your thorax and right arm. Stabilize the proximal tibia with your right hand and place your left hand on the lateral aspect of the distal femur at the joint line.

Action: Engage the motion barrier of abduction at the tibio-femoral joint. Apply a high velocity, low amplitude, medial thrust to the lateral femur. This will induce a relative lateral glide of the tibia. Reassess the range of motion and stability following the technique.

Manipulation Technique
Tibio-Femoral Joint
Medial Glide of Tibia (Relative Technique)

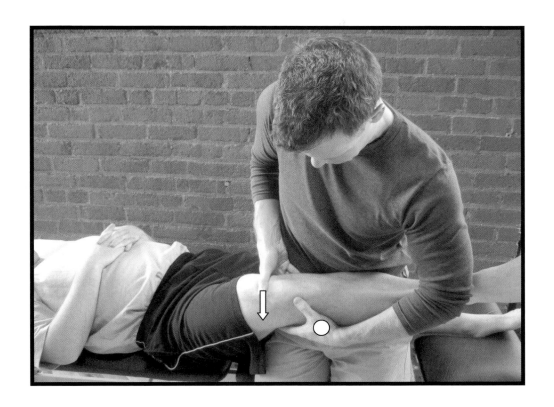

Technique described for the right tibio-femoral joint

Indication: Articular restriction of adduction

Patient: Supine with knee slightly flexed

Therapist: Standing at the side of bed with the patient's leg supported between your thorax and left arm. Stabilize the proximal tibia with your left hand and place your right hand on the medial aspect of the distal femur at the joint line.

Action: Engage the motion barrier of adduction at the tibio-femoral joint. Apply a high velocity, low amplitude, lateral thrust to the medial femur. This will induce a relative medial glide of the tibia. Reassess the range of motion and stability following the technique.

Manipulation Technique
Superior Tibio-Fibular Joint
Anterior Glide

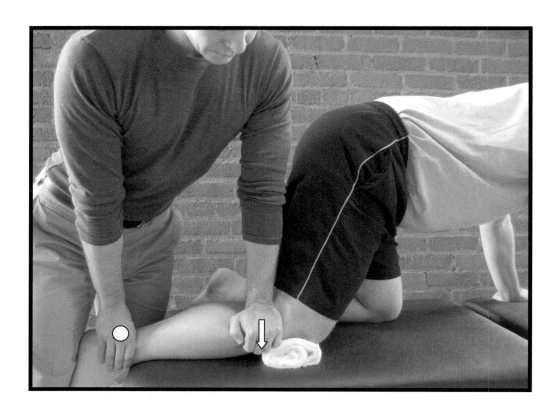

Technique described for the right superior tibio-fibular joint

Indication: Articular restriction of anterior glide

Patient: Four point kneeling with a rolled towel under knee

Therapist: Standing at the end of the bed. Stabilize the distal tibia and fibula with your right hand. Palpate the head of the fibula with the heel of your left hand.

Action: Engage the motion barrier of the anterior glide at the superior tibio-fibular joint. Apply a high velocity, low amplitude, anterior thrust to the head of the fibula. Reassess the range of motion and stability following the technique.

Manipulation Technique
Superior Tibio-Fibular Joint
Posterior Glide

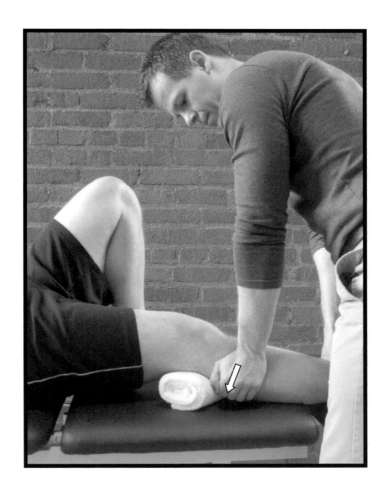

Technique described for the right superior tibio-fibular joint

Indication: Articular restriction of posterior glide

Patient: Supine with a rolled towel under knee

Therapist: Standing at the end of the bed. Stabilize the distal tibia and fibula with your right hand. Palpate the head of the fibula with the heel of your left hand.

Action: Engage the motion barrier of the posterior glide at the superior tibio-fibular joint. Apply a high velocity, low amplitude, posterior thrust to the head of the fibula. Reassess the range of motion and stability following the technique.

Manipulation Technique
Talocrural Joint
Loose Body Mobilization / Manipulation

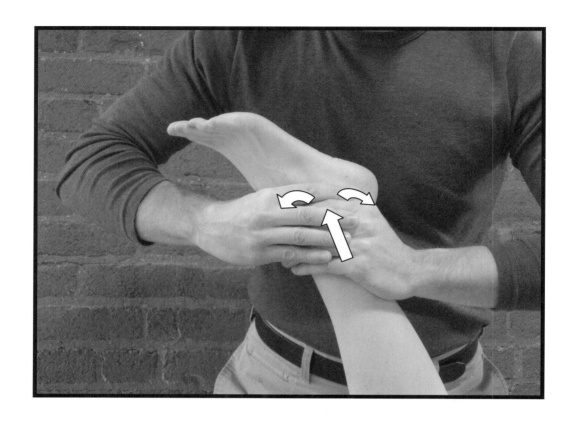

Technique described for the right talocrural joint

Indication: A loose body in the talocrural joint

Patient: Prone lying with the knee flexed

Therapist: Standing at the side of the bed. Grasp the talus with both hands.

Action: Passively assess which movement of the ankle (plantarflexion or dorsiflexion) is best tolerated by the patient. Apply a traction force to the talocrural joint while alternately flicking the patient's ankle into the movement which you found most comfortable and back to neutral. Reassess the range of motion and stability following the manipulation.

Manipulation Technique
Talocrural Joint
Traction

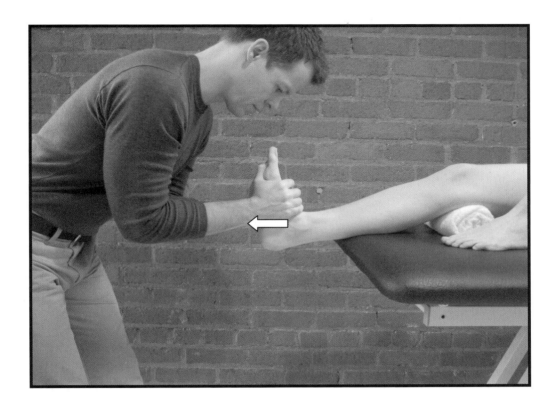

Technique described for the right ankle

Indication: Articular restriction of the talocrural joint.

Patient: Supine lying with a rolled towel under right knee and left knee flexed with foot flat on the bed

Therapist: Standing at the end of the bed with a stride stance. With both hands, grasp the patient's foot at the talocrural joint line. Keep your elbows close together.

Action: Place the talocrural joint in neutral and engage the motion barrier of traction by shifting your weight backward. Apply a high velocity, small amplitude, traction thrust to the talus. Reassess the range of motion and stability following the manipulation.

Manipulation Technique
Talocrural Joint
J-Stroke For Dorsiflexion

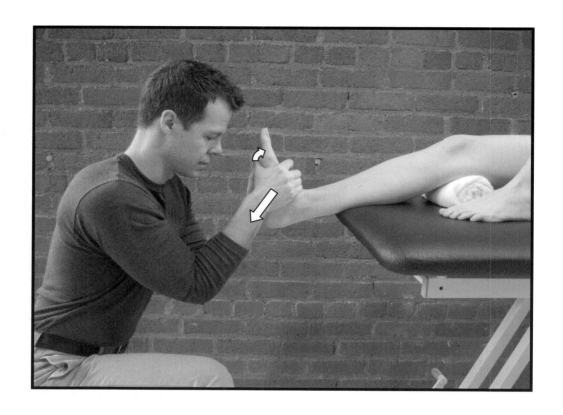

Technique described for the right ankle

Indication: Articular restriction of dorsiflexion

Patient: Supine lying with a rolled towel under right knee and left knee flexed with foot flat on the bed

Therapist: Kneeling at the end of the bed. With both hands, grasp the patient's foot at the talocrural joint line. Keep your elbows close together.

Action: Engage the motion barrier of dorsiflexion and traction by shifting your weight backward. Apply a high velocity, small amplitude, posterior-inferior thrust to the talus while keeping the talocrural joint at the limit of dorsiflexion with your thumbs. Reassess the range of motion and stability following the manipulation.

Manipulation Technique
Talocrural Joint
J-Stroke for Plantarflexion

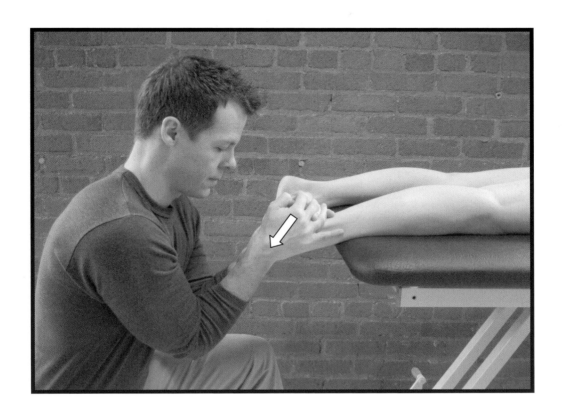

Technique described for the right ankle

Indication: Articular restriction of plantarflexion

Patient: Prone lying with foot off end of bed

Therapist: Kneeling at the end of the bed. With both hands, grasp the posterior aspect of the patient's talus and calcaneus at the talocrural joint line. Keep your elbows close together.

Action: Engage the motion barrier of plantarflexion and traction by shifting your weight backward. Apply a high velocity, small amplitude, anterior-inferior thrust to the talus. Reassess the range of motion and stability following the manipulation.

Manipulation Technique
Talocrural Joint
Anterior Glide

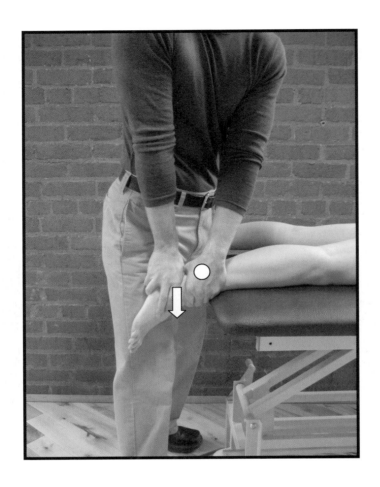

Technique described for the right ankle

Indication: Articular restriction of plantarflexion

Patient: Prone lying with foot over end of bed

Therapist: Standing at the end of the bed. Stabilize the tibia and fibula with your left hand. Grasp the posterior aspect of the talus and calcaneus with your right hand.

Action: Engage the motion barrier of plantarflexion at the talocrural joint. Apply a high velocity, small amplitude, anterior thrust to the talus. Reassess the range of motion and stability following the manipulation.

Manipulation Technique
Subtalar Joint
Loose Body Mobilization / Manipulation

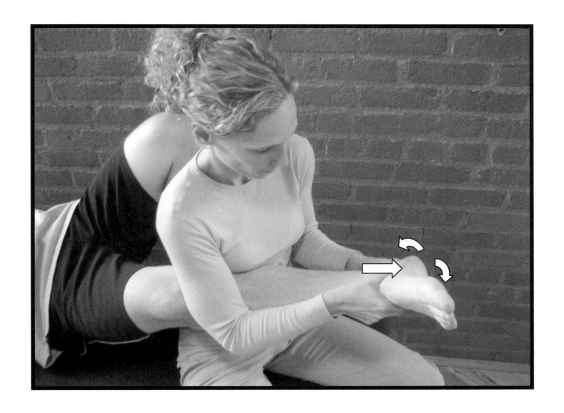

Technique described for the right subtalar joint

Indication: A loose body in the subtalar joint

Patient: Supine lying with right hip in external rotation

Therapist: Seated on the bed with the patient's leg supported between your thorax and right arm. Grasp the calcaneus with the thumbs and index fingers of both hands.

Action: Apply a traction force to the subtalar joint while simultaneously oscillating the calcaneus into pronation and supination. Reassess the range of motion and stability following the manipulation.

Manipulation Technique
Subtalar Joint
Anterior Joint Lateral Glide

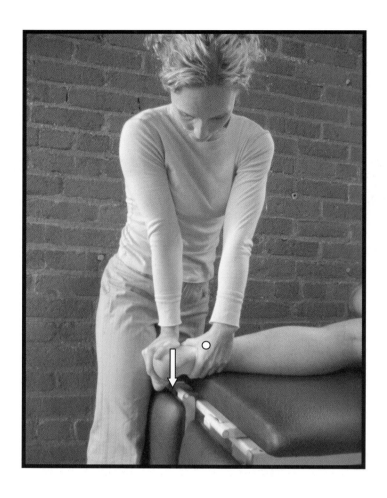

Technique described for the right subtalar joint

Indication: Articular restriction of pronation

Patient: Right side lying with foot off edge of bed

Therapist: Standing at the end of the bed. Stabilize the posterior aspect of the talus with your left hand. Place the heel of your right hand on the anterior-medial aspect of the calcaneus.

Action: Engage the motion barrier of pronation at the subtalar joint. Apply a high velocity, small amplitude, lateral thrust to the calcaneus. Reassess the range of motion and stability following the manipulation technique.

Manipulation Technique
Subtalar Joint
Anterior Joint Medial Glide

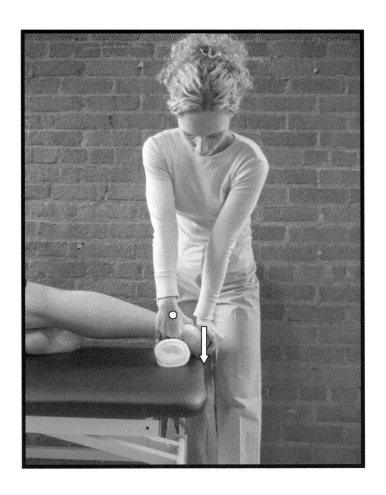

Technique described for the right subtalar joint

Indication: Articular restriction of supination

Patient: Left side lying with a rolled towel under medial malleolus

Therapist: Standing at the end of the bed. Stabilize the posterior aspect of the talus with your right hand. Place the heel of your left hand on the anterior-lateral aspect of the calcaneus.

Action: Engage the motion barrier of supination at the subtalar joint. Apply a high velocity, small amplitude, medial thrust to the calcaneus. Reassess the range of motion and stability following the manipulation technique.

Manipulation Technique
Subtalar Joint
Posterior Joint Lateral Glide

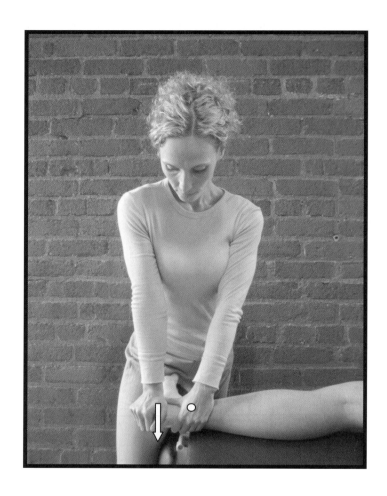

Technique described for the right subtalar joint

Indication: Articular restriction of supination

Patient: Right side lying with foot off edge of bed

Therapist: Standing at the end of the bed. Stabilize the posterior aspect of the talus with your left hand. Place the heel of your right hand on the posterior-medial aspect of the calcaneus.

Action: Engage the motion barrier of supination at the subtalar joint. Apply a high velocity, small amplitude, lateral thrust to the calcaneus. Reassess the range of motion and stability following the manipulation technique.

Manipulation Technique
Subtalar Joint
Posterior Joint Medial Glide

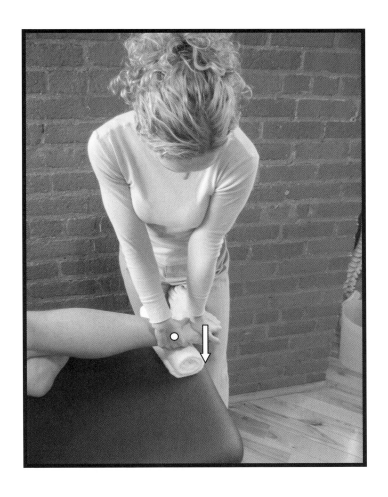

Technique described for the right subtalar joint

Indication: Articular restriction of pronation

Patient: Left side lying with a rolled towel under medial malleolus

Therapist: Standing at the end of the bed. Stabilize the posterior aspect of the talus with your right hand. Place the heel of your left hand on the posterior-lateral aspect of the calcaneus.

Action: Engage the motion barrier of pronation at the subtalar joint. Apply a high velocity, small amplitude, medial thrust to the calcaneus. Reassess the range of motion and stability following the manipulation technique.

Manipulation Technique
Subtalar Joint
Osteokinematic Flick Into Supination

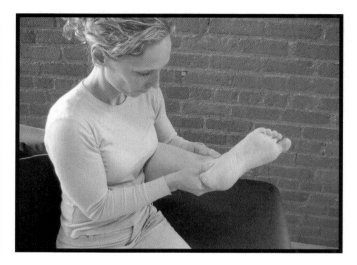

Start Position   **Finish Position**

Technique described for the right subtalar joint

Indication: Articular restriction of supination

Patient: Left side lying

Therapist: Seated at the edge of the bed supporting the patent's leg between your thorax and left arm. Stabilize the talus with the thumbs and index fingers of both hands.

Action: Apply a high velocity, small amplitude flick of the calcaneus into supination. Reassess the range of motion and stability following the manipulation technique.

Manipulation Technique
Subtalar Joint
Osteokinematic Flick Into Pronation

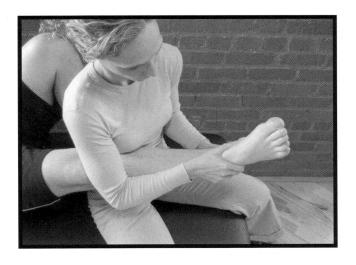

Start Position

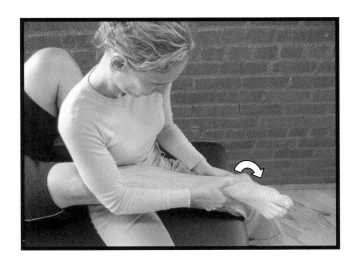

Finish Position

Technique described for the right subtalar joint

Indication: Articular restriction of pronation

Patient: Right side lying with right hip in external rotation

Therapist: Seated at the edge of the bed supporting the patent's leg between your thorax and right arm. Stabilize the talus with the thumbs and index fingers of both hands.

Action: Apply a high velocity, small amplitude flick of the calcaneus into pronation. Reassess the range of motion and stability following the manipulation technique.

Manipulation Technique
Midtarsal Joint
Traction

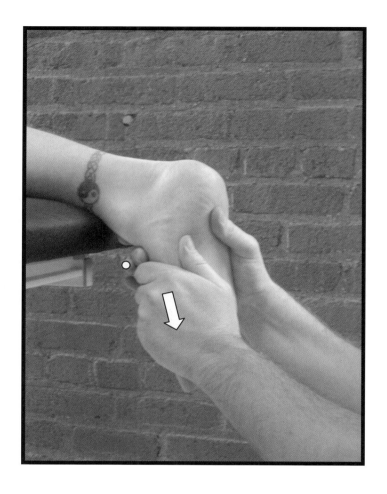

Technique described for the right talonavicular joint

Indication: Articular restriction of the midtarsal joints

Patient: Prone lying with right foot off edge of bed

Therapist: Crouched at the end of the bed. Stabilize the talus with your right hand. Grasp the navicular with your left hand.

Action: The motion barrier is engaged by taking up the slack of traction at the talonavicular joint. Apply a high velocity, small amplitude, traction thrust to the navicular. Reassess the range of motion and stability following the manipulation. This technique can be used to treat any of the midtarsal joints.

Manipulation Technique
Talonavicular Joint
Plantar Glide

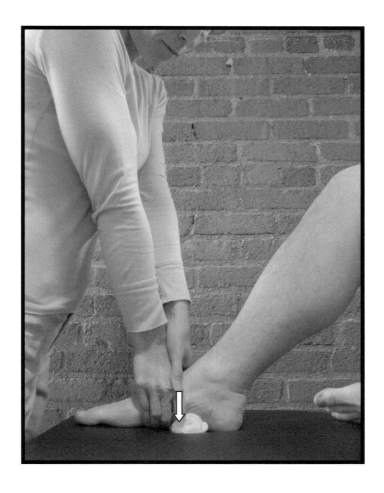

Technique described for the right talonavicular joint

Indication: Articular restriction of supination

Patient: Crook lying with a rolled face cloth under the head of the talus

Therapist: Standing at the end of the bed. Place your right second metacarpophalangeal joint over the dorsal aspect of the navicular. Reinforce your right hand with your left hand.

Action: Engage the motion barrier of supination. Apply a high velocity, small amplitude, plantar thrust to the navicular. Reassess the range of motion and stability following the manipulation.

Manipulation Technique
Talonavicular Joint
Dorsal Glide

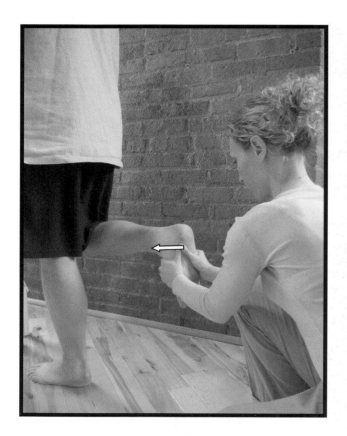 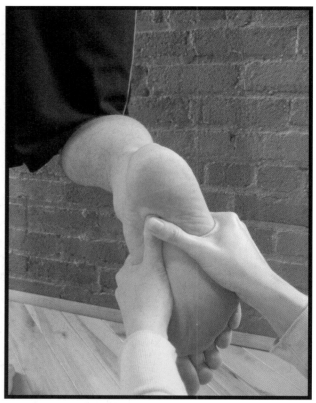

Technique described for the right talonavicular joint

Indication: Articular restriction of pronation

Patient: Standing with hand on bed for balance with right knee flexed

Therapist: Crouching behind the patient. Grasp the foot with both hands and dorsiflex the talocrural joint. Place your left thumb on the plantar aspect of the navicular and overlap with your right thumb. Take care not to block the navicular with your fingers anteriorly.

Action: Engage the motion barrier of pronation. Apply a high velocity, small amplitude, dorsal thrust to the navicular. Take care not to plantarflex the foot as you apply your manipulation. Reassess the range of motion and stability following the manipulation.

Manipulation Technique
Calcaneocuboid Joint
Plantar Glide

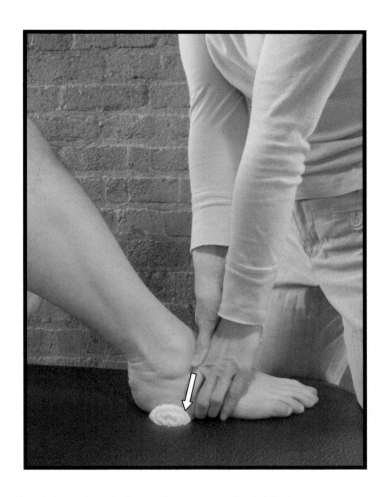

Technique described for the right calcaneocuboid joint

Indication: Articular restriction of supination

Patient: Crook lying with a rolled face cloth under the distal calcaneus

Therapist: Standing at the end of the bed. Place your left second metacarpophalangeal joint over the dorsal aspect of the cuboid. Reinforce your left hand with your right hand.

Action: Engage the motion barrier of supination. Apply a high velocity, small amplitude, plantar thrust to the cuboid. Reassess the range of motion and stability following the manipulation.

Manipulation Technique
Calcaneocuboid Joint
Dorsal Glide

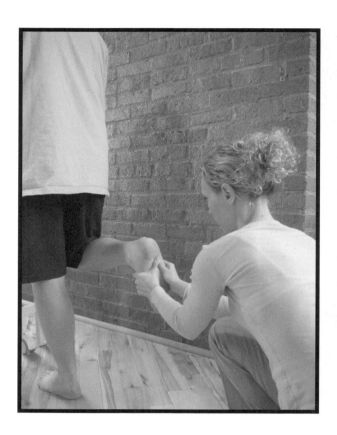 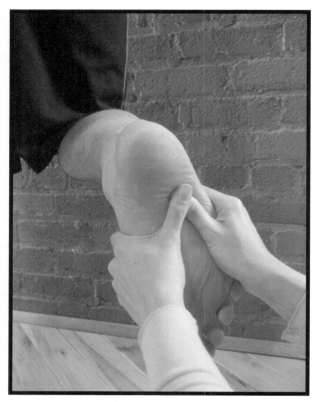

Technique described for the right calcaneocuboid joint

Indication: Articular restriction of pronation

Patient: Standing with hand on bed for balance with right knee flexed

Therapist: Crouching behind the patient. Grasp the foot with both hands and dorsiflex the talocrural joint. Place your right thumb on the plantar aspect of the cuboid and overlap with your thumb. Take care not to block the cuboid with your fingers anteriorly.

Action: Engage the motion barrier of pronation. Apply a high velocity, small amplitude, dorsal thrust to the cuboid. Take care not to plantarflex the foot as you apply your manipulation. Reassess the range of motion and stability following the manipulation

Manipulation Technique
Cuneonavicular Joint
Plantar Glide

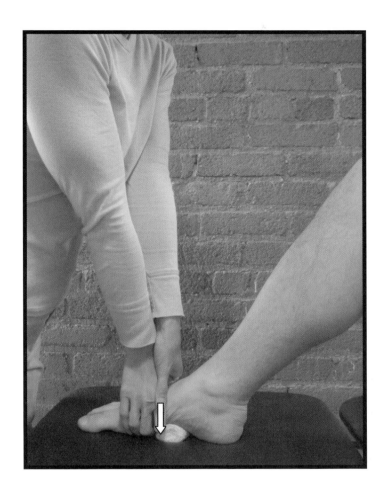

Technique described for the right medial cuneonavicular joint

Indication: Articular restriction of supination

Patient: Crook lying with a rolled face cloth under the head of the talus

Therapist: Standing at the end of the bed. Place your right second metacarpophalangeal joint over the dorsal aspect of the medial cuneiform. Reinforce your right hand with your left hand.

Action: Engage the motion barrier of supination. Apply a high velocity, small amplitude, plantar thrust to the medial cuneiform. Reassess the range of motion and stability following the manipulation.

Manipulation Technique
Cuneonavicular Joint
Dorsal Glide

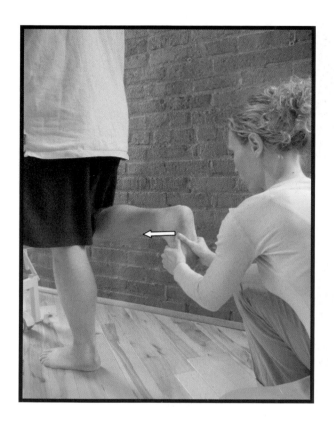 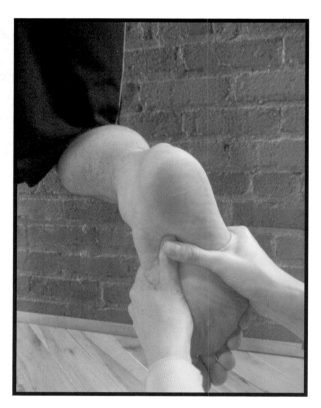

Technique described for the right medial cuneonavicular joint

Indication: Articular restriction of pronation

Patient: Standing with hand on bed for balance with right knee flexed

Therapist: Crouching behind the patient. Grasp the foot with both hands and dorsiflex the talocrural joint. Place your left thumb on the plantar aspect of the medial cuneiform and overlap with your right thumb. Take care not to block the medial cuneiform with your fingers anteriorly.

Action: Engage the motion barrier of pronation. Apply a high velocity, small amplitude, dorsal thrust to the medial cuneiform. Take care not to plantarflex the foot as you apply your manipulation. Reassess the range of motion and stability following the manipulation. This technique can be adapted to treat the other cuneiform bones.

Manipulation Technique
TMT Joint
Traction

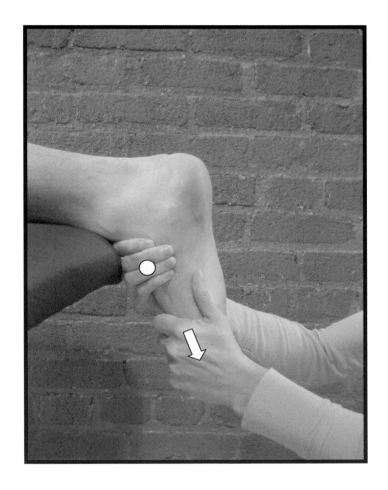

Technique described for the right first TMT joint

Indication: Articular restriction of the first TMT joint

Patient: Prone lying with right foot off edge of bed

Therapist: Crouching at the end of the bed. Stabilize the first medial cuneiform with your right hand. Grasp the first metatarsal with your left index finger and thumb.

Action: Engage the motion barrier of traction at the first TMT joint. Apply a high velocity, small amplitude, traction thrust to the first metatarsal. Reassess the range of motion and stability following the manipulation. This technique can be repeated for the first to fifth TMT joints.

Manipulation Technique
MTP and IP Joints
Traction

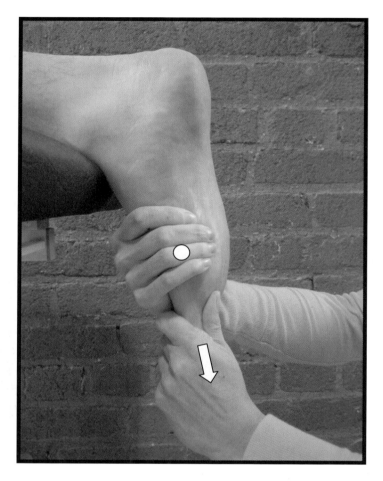

Technique described for the right first MTP joint

Indication: Articular restriction of the first MTP joint

Patient: Prone lying with right foot off edge of bed

Therapist: Crouching at the end of the bed. Stabilize the first metatarsal with your right hand. Grasp the first proximal phalanx with your left index finger and thumb.

Action: Engage the motion barrier of traction at the first MTP joint. Apply a high velocity, small amplitude, traction thrust to the proximal phalanx. Reassess the range of motion and stability following the manipulation. This technique can be repeated for the second to fifth MTP joints and the first to fifth IP joints.

Manipulation Technique
Lumbar Spine
Unilateral Oblique Distraction Manipulation (Gap)

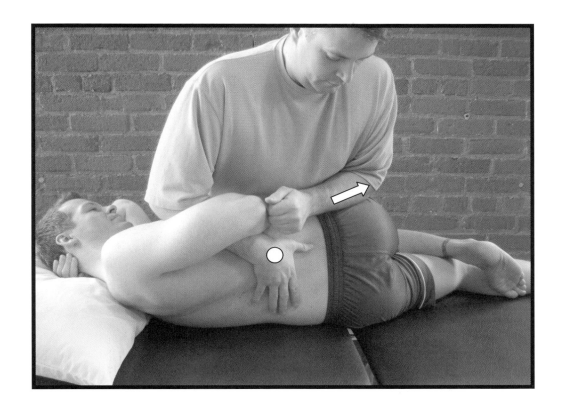

Technique described for the right L4-5 segment

Indication: Unilateral articular restriction of flexion or extension in the lumbar spine

Patient: Left side lying at the edge of the bed

Therapist: Standing at the side of the bed. Lock the patient from above and below, leaving L4-5 in neutral. Place your right arm under the patient's right arm and stabilize it against the thorax with your right hip. Palpate the spinous process of L4 with your right hand. Place your left forearm on the patient's iliac crest.

Action: Engage the motion barrier of L4-5. Apply a high velocity, low amplitude, anterior-inferior thrust to the patient's pelvis. Reassess the range of motion and stability following the manipulation.

Manipulation Technique
Lumbar Spine
Unilateral Extension Manipulation

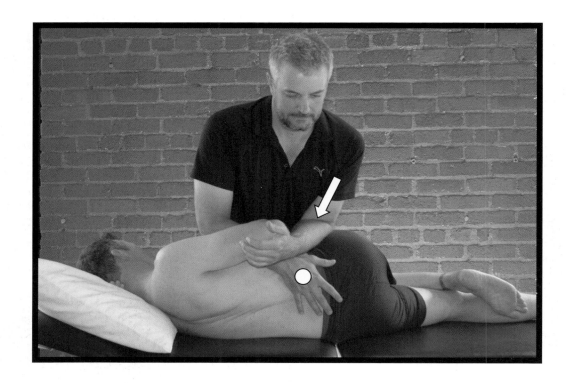

Technique described for the right L4-5 segment

Indication: Unilateral articular restriction of extension in the lumbar spine

Patient: Left side lying at the edge of the bed

Therapist: Standing at the side of the bed. Lock the patient from above and below, leaving L4-5 in neutral. Place your right arm under the patient's right arm and lightly stabilize it against the thorax with your right hip. Palpate the spinous process of L4 with your right hand. Place your left forearm on the patient's iliac crest.

Action: Engage the motion barrier of extension at L4-5. Apply a high velocity, low amplitude, superior / anterior thrust to the patient's pelvis. Reassess the range of motion and stability following the manipulation.

Manipulation Technique
SI Joint
Supine Distraction

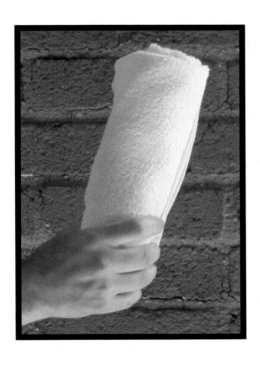

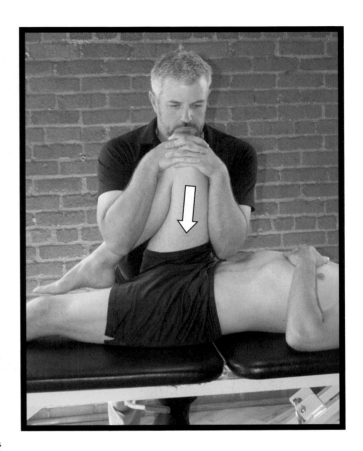

Technique described for the right SI joint

Indication: Unilateral articular restriction of the sacroiliac joint

Patient: Supine lying at the edge of the bed

Therapist: Standing at the side of the bed. Place a rolled towel medial to the patient's right PSIS on the sacral sulcus. With the patient's hip at 90 degrees, place both hands on the right knee with an interlock grip. Align your forearms along the long axis of the femur.

Action: Take up the motion in the hip joint by using combinations of hip flexion / adduction / internal rotation. Engage the motion barrier by applying a posterior directed force to the patient's femur using a combination of your body and arms. Apply a high velocity, low amplitude posterior thrust to the patient's pelvis through the femur. Reassess the range of motion and stability following the manipulation.

Manipulation Technique
SI Joint
Supine Inferior Thrust

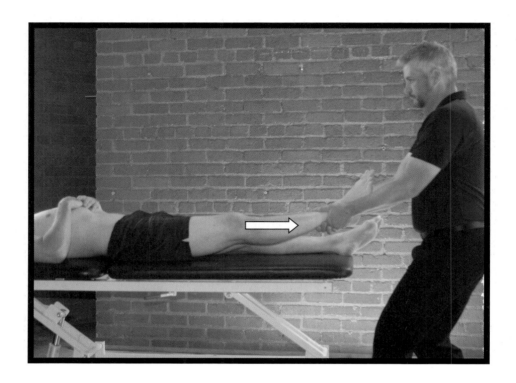

Technique described for the right SI joint

Indication: Unilateral superior articular fixation of the sacroiliac joint. This is the preferred technique if the SI joint fixation includes posterior rotation of the innominate.

Patient: Supine lying

Therapist: Standing at the end of the bed. With both hands grasp the patient's leg just above the malleoli. Try to align your forearms in the same direction as you want to thrust.

Action: Engage the motion barrier by applying an inferior force to the patient's leg by leaning back gently with your body. Apply a high velocity, low amplitude, inferior thrust to the patient's pelvis through the leg with your arms. Reassess the range of motion and stability following the manipulation.

Manipulation Technique
SI Joint
Prone Inferior Thrust

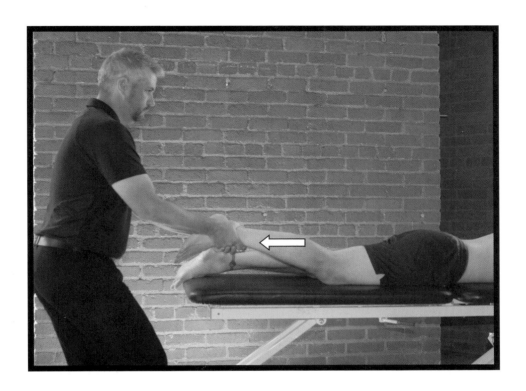

Technique described for the right SI joint

Indication: Unilateral superior articular fixation of the sacroiliac joint. This is the preferred technique if the SI joint fixation includes anterior rotation of the innominate.

Patient: Prone lying with hands crossed under their head.

Therapist: Standing at the end of the bed. With both hands grasp the patient's leg just above the malleoli. Try to align your forearms in the same direction as you want to thrust.

Action: Engage the motion barrier by applying an inferior force to the patient's leg by leaning back gently with your body. Apply a high velocity, low amplitude, inferior thrust to the patient's pelvis through the leg with your arms. Reassess the range of motion and stability following the manipulation.

References

Canadian Physiotherapy Association, Orthopaedic Division Advanced Manual and Manipulative Therapy Course Curriculum

Canadian Physiotherapy Association, Orthopaedic Division Advanced Manual and Manipulative Therapy Level System Manuals 1 to 5

Lee D 2004, The Pelvic Girdle, Third Ed. Churchill and Livingstone, Edinburgh

Nolan M, Walsh M, Clinical Assessment and Treatment Techniques for the Lower Extremity, Canada 1997